A story of love, loss, and forgiveness

WHY DO DOGS DIE?

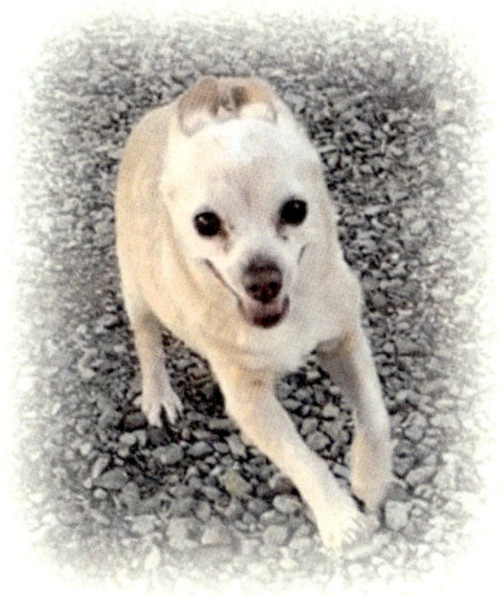

By Mikki Moon Star

(Mikki L. Padilla)

The information the author shares in this book is based on personal recollections, interactions, situations, observations, conversations, energy exchanges, and accounts of events of her own experiences and the manner in which they occurred. Every effort was made to corroborate memory with fact for the personal experiences stated; those experiences are as true as the author could make them. Some names have been changed and events compressed.

This book details the journey that connected the author back with dogs, her mission, and to a place of embracing their transitions and all endings. The information is not intended to cause loss, damage, or disruption to any person, place, business, organization, or animal discussed inside. The intent of the author is to provide personal information that is of a healing, loving, inspirational nature in order to help you in your quest for emotional, physical, and spiritual well-being.

ISBN: 9798-218-13553-9

Independently published

Book Cover Design by Edgar Flores
www.eflo-art.com

Book Cover Modifications by Fitzgerald Munoz
Book's Interior Images Edited by Fitzgerald Munoz
www.fitzmunozphoto.com

Book Cover Modifications by Scott Gerber
Scott Gerber Design
(In loving memory)

Furever Soulmates
www.FureverSoulmates.com

Love and Gratitude To:

Fitzgerald Munoz
Edgar Flores
Scott Gerber
Chris Jr.
Erin Hiser
Janet Linden
Pamela Gregg Flax
My Soul Lighting Friends and Healers
Animal Lovers, Adopters, Fosters, Networkers, Volunteers, and Rescuers
Bodhi, Lola, Dipper, Cosmo, Spirit, Digo, Charly, Tippet, Rudy, Fritz & Peaches
All the animals and creatures I've been blessed to help have better lives
My Furever Connective Pet Family
All Beloved Pets of My Parents Through Time
My Beautiful Parents
Goldie

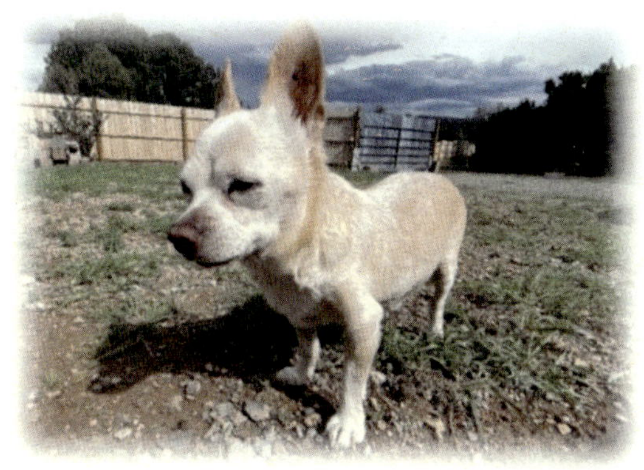

My beautiful Little Dipper "Veteran" Moon. Whatever cosmic realm you're enjoying to the fullest, I know that you're in your highest light, happiest, and healthiest. I miss and love you more than anything. And although I am pained without you, I am happy for you. I want to thank you for choosing me – and for coming into my life – and giving me such meaning and purpose, especially at a time when I needed it, and you, the most. Your soul was so gentle, soft, and fragile. Yet, you were resilient and robust as ever. Strong was an understatement, even though some days your body got sick too. You brought me back to what was truly important and taught me how to live and love like every day was my last. You also showed me the significance of not giving anything heavy too much attention. Because so, I'm able to let go of attachments. I learned not to be in such a hurry and that there's no point in turning back. I knew we'd be together for 'our' ever from the moment I met you. It was love at first sight. How lucky was I to have shared such depth with you? Nothing else mattered, but you. I am so glad that I never missed a single second of your progress, aura, personality, enthusiasm, or breath. Down to your very last, I am so grateful that I was holding you close. I am such a better person since you, and I will cherish our time together for eternity. From the sun to the moon, the air to the ocean, the sky to the soil... we are rooted together forever in our souls. You are my kin... my oxygen... my everything. And because of you my dear little warrior... the rescues will go on!

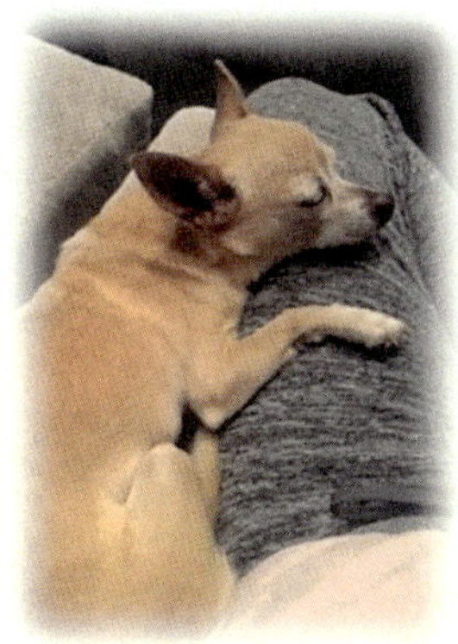

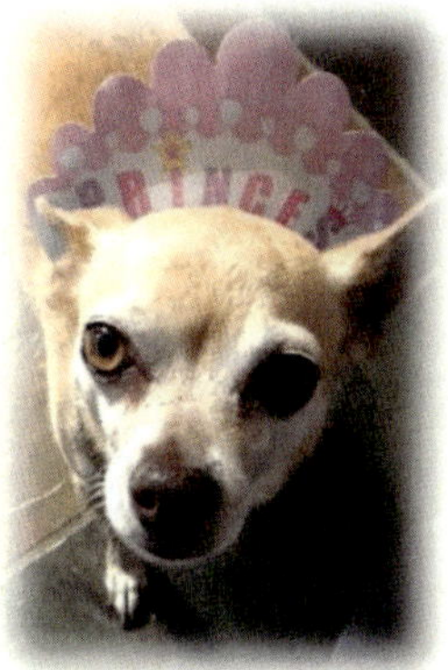

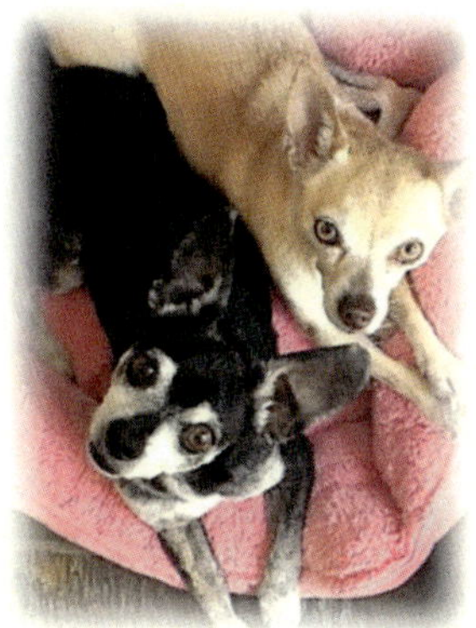

My darling Charly. There aren't enough words to describe your beautiful soul... and how deeply you touched mine. Everything about you was pure love and energy in the most abundant form. You were filled with gentleness, confidence, playfulness, compassion, wisdom, empathy, and the type of unconditional devotion that people dream about. From the moment I entered your world, I knew you were a special little girl. How lucky was I to be able to connect with the brightest part of your light?! It's been unbelievably painful not to have spent the rest of your life with you and Tippet. Yet, you've both been forever engrained in my heart, thoughts, and decisions, fused in my spirit, and will always show up in every rescue that I continue to rescue. It was because of you that I went on to help extend the quality of life for forgotten pets. Since we were separated, there has never been a day that I didn't miss you guys more than the day before. Thank goodness I see the preciousness of your eyes by the way Bodhi stares into mine, and how he grabs me with his paws so that I'll never let go (just like you used to do). I can't wait to cuddle close with you again, roll over and do stretchies, rub tummies, give kissies, watch you smudge your face in the wet grass, meditate with our crystals, gaze at the fishies swimming in the river, play with Little Duckie, go for endless walks, hikes, and rides, share yummy treats, never leave one another's side, and tell each other every second of every single day, "*I love you.*" Until then, I know you'll keep watching over Tippet and protect him like you always did. If he's already joined you, then please give him tons of smooches and tight hugs for me, and tell him that I miss him dearly. Thank you for such a loving experience, my princess. Enjoy paradise to the fullest!

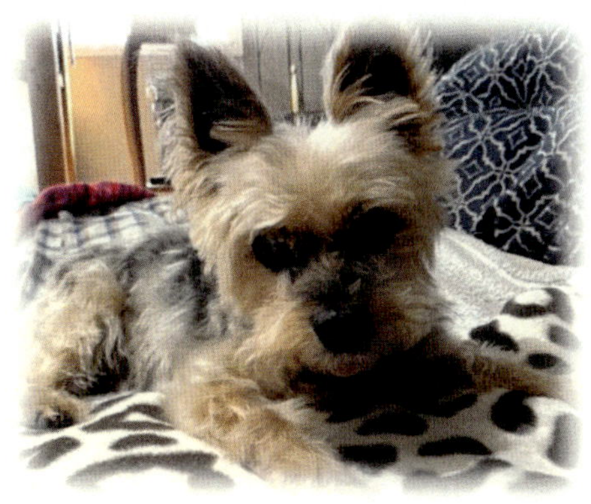

My precious Cosmo. How did I get so lucky to share life with you, be trusted by you, loved by you, and connected on all levels with you? Never did I think I'd be blessed with another soulmate again, and so soon. From the second I saw your photo, I knew you found me. From the instant we met, I knew we were meant to be. We began our journey one foot, feel, and vibe at a time... as your senses grasped your new environment in ways I hadn't experienced. From so many supposed ailments, you my love, healed the fastest!!! I saw your life and confidence illuminate by the way your silky hair grew back, how you put healthy weight on, sniffed things out differently, dug and played in your blankies, raced through the yard where you were initially skeptic, meditated in the beaming sun rays on the bedroom floor, enjoyed the breeze blowing through your pores, grounded as we went earthing and, most of all, our side-by-side cuddling. You were such a treasure to grow with, learn from, and be reminded of how valuable the present moment was. I hadn't ever encountered such a delicate, sweet, little unique soul with so much zest and courageousness. You appreciated absolutely everything, and it was so beautifully fulfilling. They say that your heart dogs will send you another dog to carry on the love story and life course. That, my little Cozzy, you surely were. I'll never understand why our last day turned out the way it did, and certainly not the short span of time I got with you. But I will take with me the gratefulness for life that you retaught me and the unconditional bond you shared with me... and hang on to all other days we spent close together making forever memories. I love and miss you more than ever. I'm so glad you finally appeared in my dreams to show me that you're okay, and still filled with the purest of love, innocence, and sweetness in every way!

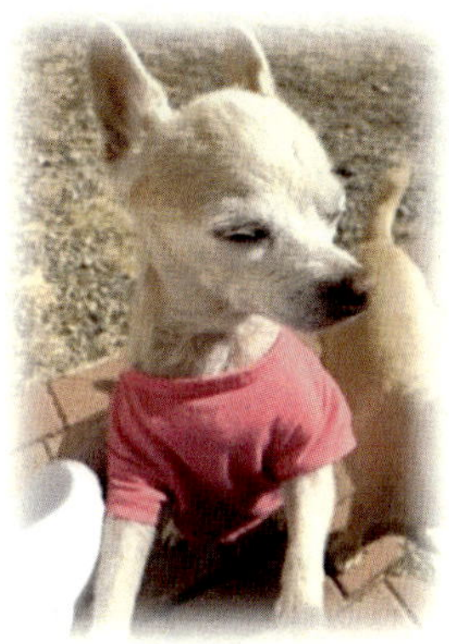 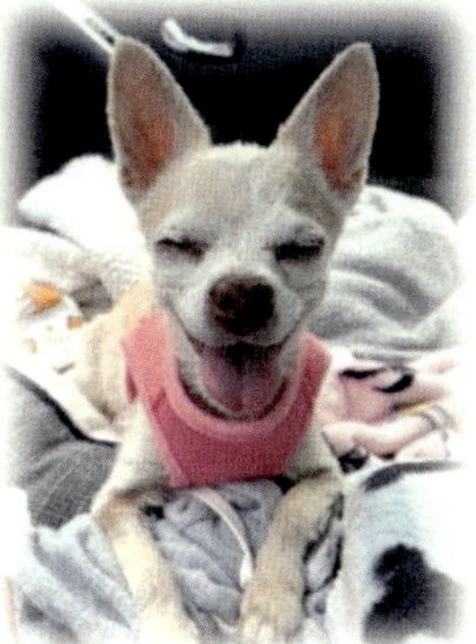 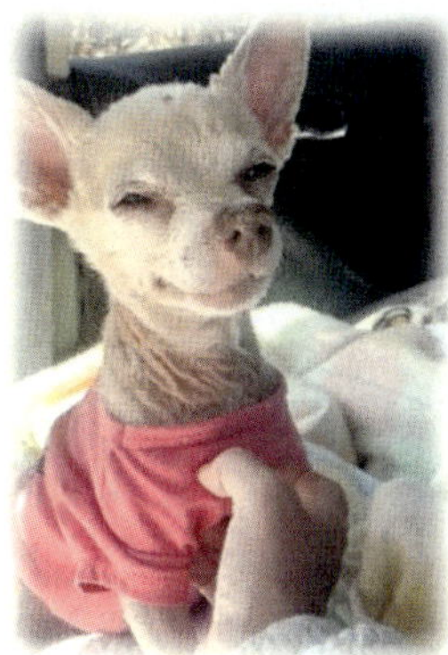

Spirit Moon… my greatest love of all. What a gift it was to exchange pure harmony with the prettiest soul in the prettiest doggy body. You were my furever from the very beginning. Like two flowers blossoming together, we were a reflection and extension of each other. Everywhere we walked, drove, laid, cuddled, ate, and just sat in silence… I could see my heart beating outside of my body in the form of you. I loved watching how safe, comfortable, and confident you felt. And even more, how treasured and loved you knew you were. I don't know life without you as it has been airless in your absence. The light in my soul has temporarily dimmed. This part of true love is the hardest. I loved you the most… lived, learned, and was happiest with you the most. That's why it hurts the most. You were such a darling goddess filled with softness, fun, trust, strength, openness, consciousness, and connected to all things possible and wonderful. I'm sure gonna miss being inseparable with you – traveling the property path with you – seeing you in your corner spot on top of the couch – kissing you a million times a day – holding you close while licking my face – driving with you on my lap while taking in the views – making you amazing meals – your passion for food and treats – watching you walk up the pillow steps to the bed – sleeping right next to me – your radiant smile and bright eyes – deep snore – awesome bark – adorable howl – cute outfits – rolling on your back – giving you baths – meditating – daily massages – and enjoying bones to the fullest. You were my everything, and all that restored my organ back to wellness. I'm so blessed that you chose me to live out the rest of your beautiful life with. Thank goodness for the thousands of photos and videos I have of you to continually relive the best 478 days of my own. My love for you will always be infinite, my happy little pink moon!

CONTENTS

PART 1

Not Every Love Story Has a Beautiful Beginning

1
The Root

For the first sixteen years of my spiritual growth, I was blessed to have animals share their hearts with me. But I'd go on to spend almost thirty more missing out on that incredible companionship. From my teens to age forty-three, I was too busy thinking that I knew where I wanted to go and who I wanted to be. I was young, athletic, scholastic, and personable, with the spark to take on the world. I didn't have any idea what I was doing. But I had been bullied since elementary school, so my pathway was already taking shape.

Early on, I found myself to be more of a one-on-one person without needing to be in large groups. I was better equipped and inclined to hang out with boys over girls, and fiercely independent in action and in thought. You could say that I was developing as an "outside of the box" type of pundit. I'm not quite sure if the persistence to be successful was in my blood, or that it was just a way to escape and feel important. If anything, that determination kept me occupied enough to lessen how often I got picked on.

The kids I associated with had their own unique gifts, strengths, and levels of amazement. We all somewhat had visions early on and looked to pursue different ambitions. Yet, I felt like the way of life among similar economic households leaned more on getting married at an early age, having kids, and either working for the city or staying home raising their young. I made no judgments regarding the patterns of a small-town environment, but it just didn't resonate with me. I always felt like there was so much more out there to venture into and be a part of. I didn't have any idea what was in store for my future. Yet, I didn't care. That was probably due to having parents and a few teachers that instilled me with positive reinforcement and an open belief system to help catapult my talents. I just found myself never able to grasp a single permanent goal that would carry me through the next three decades.

Over the years, it became clear that I was never one of those people that knew what I wanted to do for the rest of my life by the time I reached age six. You'd hear of athletes that honed in on their dreams of pitching in the big leagues by kindergarten, and doctors, teachers, and actors working on their craft in their backyards with their pretend patients and stages. It seemed like things just came to me, so I went with what I was good at in the temporary moment. And that was primarily sports, math, writing, and science. I did, however, think I'd be a superstar and a veterinarian by the fourth grade. What an unlikely mix of goals. I was very charismatic and knew that I could light up any room. I also had a fond love for animals.

We lived a couple of streets over from an arroyo. So, on days when some of the guys and I weren't jumping the banks on our motor-cycles, we would ride our peddle bikes to the same areas and catch horny toads and lizards. Then, as the seasons changed and the rain fell, I'd go find tadpoles in the puddles. My intent was to give them better homes. But obviously, captivation of any life form was not the right course of action. I was a kid, so I guess I had to learn through my own experimentation. I must say that I had quite a cool reptile display on my back porch along with my bunny's 5-star luxurious cabana. Her cushioned cage provided her with warmth, comfort, and safety when she wasn't out enjoying the spacious quarter acre of green grass. My assemble of beloveds sure did bring me fulfillment.

My parents encouraged interaction and involvement with creatures of different classifications. The only problem was that I really hadn't learned how to take care of them. I was sure that I could figure it out, but had no idea of the indirect trauma that would develop from those experiences. I had a few tadpoles dry up and my rabbit got mauled by a next-door dog after leaving her out in the yard to freely roam around. I never thought anything would happen in the two hours I went to the movies. That would be the first of my funerals.

Fortunately, I still had my two amazing doggies who stood by my side through my many lessons and attempts. I don't recall how "Fritz" and "Peaches" came into my life. I just remember how much I loved them by age five. Peaches was a fluffy gorgeous white miniature Poodle and Fritz was a silky copper purebred miniature Dachshund.

Oh, the fun I had with those dogs. We would color in our Crayola books and, almost every time, Peaches would end up green. We'd play fetch out in the backyard and Fritz would show us how fast his short little legs were. We'd pick crab-apples from our trees while both dogs awaited the homemade pies that would come from them. We would eat treats together, snuggle together, and go fishing and camping together. On many occasions, I'd be tubing down the river only to come back and find them both layered in shit from rolling around in cow patties. Those two were just as daring as I was and relished in the excitement they could create while in the middle of nature. We were best friends and, as we grew connectively and collectively, our best parts merged with each other.

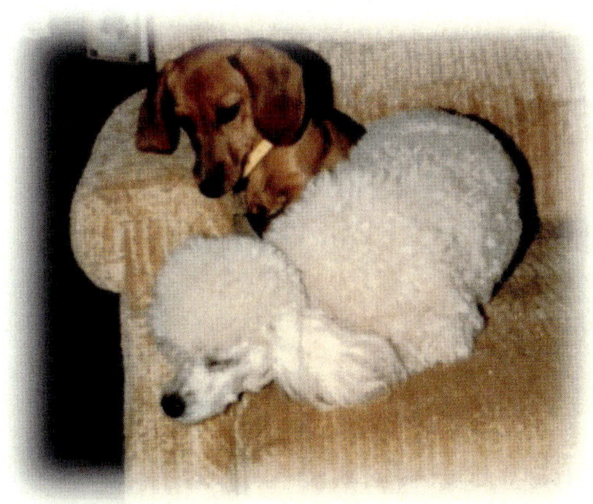

One time my parents had a party and I had to make sure they were safely away from the guests. Fritz and Peaches were such friendly beings, but we couldn't take a chance that someone would get too drunk and leave a door open for them to get out. I always allowed them to stay in my bedroom. But for some reason, I placed their cushions and blankets in the pantry. I didn't know if any of the adults were going to bring their kids to the party for me to play with, so I wanted to keep them close just in case we had to create our own fun. I knew I was probably only going to last about twenty-five minutes before I got bored around the adults anyway. I'd have just enough time to dig into the appetizers and then head back to the pantry so that we could continue playing.

Like clockwork, my internal bell rang twenty-five minutes later and I returned to check on them. When I slid the door open, both dogs were laboring to breathe while sprawled out on the floor. I didn't know if they were dead. There were open bags of chocolate chips right next to them. Somehow, they had tugged the bags down from the bottom shelf and ate most of the contents. My poor dogs were in shock! They had eaten an enormous amount of chocolate. How in the world could I have let that happen? I don't remember if the party stopped or if we took them to the animal hospital. I just had an awful feeling that I almost killed my own pets. Fortunately, they both survived and fully recovered. But that event would spiral into hidden psychological damage stuffed somewhere deep in my system.

I adored Fritz and Peaches, and all my other animals and creatures, but still managed to be careless with my priorities. I didn't pick up poop, didn't take them for walks, and didn't make sure they were supplied with food and water. I left that all up to my parents, who also had careers, bills, and problems of their own. They still had to raise me and transport me back and forth from all the activities I was involved in.

I quickly became one of those kids who only had time for my dogs when they were puppies, but less time as they got older. I know, I was just a child, right? Puppies were so cute and, at that time in society, I had no idea about shelters or sanctuaries. We never adopted or rescued. Even though I don't remember how Fritz and Peaches came into my life, I can bet that we found them at the pet shop. Until I could take on the responsibilities of the ones I had, there would be no more additions. Then, before I knew it, my dad had rehomed the both of them. I remembered being so distraught and heartbroken. Just like that, my dogs were gone and I couldn't understand why.

He would explain later that it was his way of showing me how big of a job it was to take care of a pet, and how important it was to make them number one. I felt it to be a punishment and a series of life classes wrapped together in order to teach me that dogs were living beings who were very much part of the family. As simple as he could make it, he told me that life wasn't always about fun and games. Dogs weren't toys. I couldn't just drop them off and leave them when I was done playing with them. I couldn't take them back to the store if they didn't fit or do what I wanted. I'd have to pick up shit and sacrifice time to make sure they were loved, protected, and well-cared for. Then he reminded me that they were a 100% dependent on us.

I gulped down my guilt and regret with the last bit of my saliva, and realized that they didn't deserve my lack of treatment. After several silent seconds, my dad softened his tone in a way he knew how to connect with me. He let me know that it wasn't wrong to be a growing kid who was too busy in life not to be able to dedicate the time and space for a pet. What was wrong was knowing that and still having one. My dad kept it realer than real. I was terribly hurt in hearing those words, and even more pained knowing that I'd never see my dogs again. But I had to admit that it was the beginning of waking up.

When families are so caught up in developing every piece of their blood unit, who has the time to adequately take care of pets? Not many. Instead, those animals stay home all day, alone, and only become important when they are convenient. That was me as a kid. I know I never meant it to be that way. But as upsetting as it is to hear me speak about it, that was a part of my truth.

It wasn't but a year or two later that my dad would give me the chance to try again. And I failed again. He didn't waste any time in giving the little puppy a better place to live. He rehomed my third dog in three years as I hadn't been a responsible pet sibling or caretaker. It took some time for me to think that I grasped the loss. Maybe I did because, somehow, I got back to other activities. I had to. I was an athlete and in the top tier of my educational studies. I had afterschool practice for the sport of that season, and on to two hours of cleaning office buildings with my dad for my own personal source of income. Dinner and homework followed. That was the wonder of the Universe: it forced me to pay attention to something else, even when I was 8 years old and had no idea how it all worked.

I don't know what came over my dad, but within months of my third rehoming of a pet, he thought he'd give it one last shot. Just maybe, I'd finally understand the importance of another living soul and the obligation I had to their well-being. He surprised me one day with a tiny jet-black purebred Pomeranian puppy. The little dude was electrical and had an abundance of compassion in his eyes. It was definitely love at first sight. I named him "Rudy" and he immediately became my everything. We played, ran around, investigated the huge yard, and gazed into the sunlight while holding each other tight. We cuddled close, ate our food side by side, took drives together, played kickball together, and had a blast chasing the basketball together.

He was such a jovial little dog. Seeing him live so freely was amazing. I knew he could never replace Fritz or Peaches. They would have their own story along my timeline and two of the most special spots in my heart. At such a young age, I had already begun to perceive them as my guides in the way that I would treat and care for Rudy. I vowed to never again make any dog feel less than important. Rudy was a new narration in a new chapter with a new start. All I could do was put my pencil to the paper and try again in hopes that I finally learned the value of animals. I already loved him to the planets. There was no way I was going to let him down.

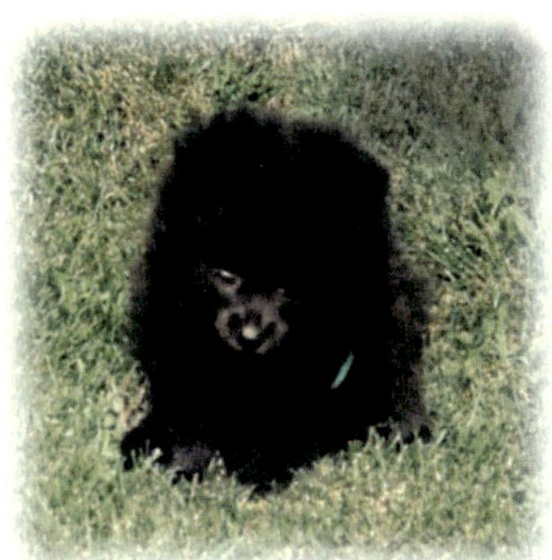

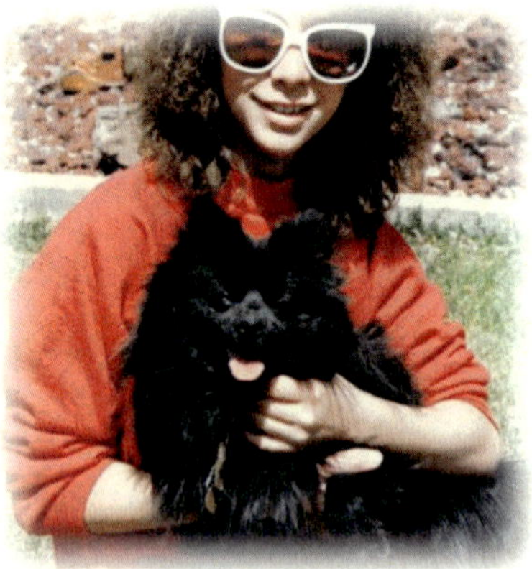

My parents separated four years after getting Rudy and, although they remained best friends, I stayed living with my dad. We ended up moving up the street to a less expensive rental home with a much smaller yard, so Rudy experienced a bit of shock. There was no grass; only concrete and gravel. It was much different than the quarter acre backyard with trees and green lawn. I felt so badly for him, but I still spent all the time I could with him. I was getting older though, and our energy shared together would become less frequent.

I entered my teens, which meant a new school, sports, activities, and interests. My dad had been a stay-at-home parent due to a disabling heart condition. So, luckily, he was always with Rudy. Then came high school and a new layer of attractions transpired. I was on top of the world socially, athletically, and scholastically. I could've never envisioned such a superstar year, especially since spending so many previous getting harassed. Then in April of that final semester, I broke the center metacarpal in my left hand from diving into a fence to catch a foul ball. It was the first inning of a fast-pitched softball game in which I heard scouts were in the stands. If that was the case, then I sure did give them a show for the first three outs, but became sidelined for another four weeks.

Not but seven days after having my cast removed and two weeks from finishing my freshman year, I got into a horrible automobile accident. It was the middle of the night and I was coming back from a college graduation in Colorado. Suddenly, a 700-pound Black Bear began to cross the interstate. He had been eating a dead rotted elk carcass. My dad was driving the truck in front while I was following close behind in another truck with my boyfriend. My dad instantly swerved to the left as he tried to avoid hitting the animal, but ended up side swiping it. Before we knew it, our vehicle slammed into the bear, then veered off to the left side of the highway. The truck rolled over several times and then landed upright among a debris of dust. The top of the cab pinned my boyfriend over the steering wheel, whereas I was ejected approximately fifty feet. I had been stretched out on the front seat sleeping, so I wasn't locked into my safety belt.

After waiving down some passers, they and my dad found me lying face down in a cluster of Chamizo bushes. We were in the middle of the mountains with no streetlights, cops, or sirens. When the paramedics arrived, they swiveled me over onto my back so that I was faced upward. My mouth was jammed with glass, my left arm was contorted around my neck, and my frame was twisted.

The first responders rushed me to the nearest hospital where it was determined that I had sustained a multitude of seemingly life-threatening injuries. I had broken my back in two places as two of my vertebrae were crushed, my left scapula was cracked, my right elbow was extrovertedly dislocated, I had a skull fracture to the back of my head, I was bleeding out of my ears, and had a blow to my pancreas. It was believed that my shoulders and coccyx were compressed like a sandwich when I was ejected. In turn, it mashed the Thoracic area of my spinal column. Half of the right side of my face was ripped off, and many of my teeth were either knocked out or cracked, and imbedded in my gums. The rest of my body was ravished with deep lacerations. Talk about a path change from everything I had ever dreamt of. Fortunately, I didn't remember a single thing about that car crash other than the pain of the aftermath. Otherwise, it could've been drastically worse.

Recovery meant zero bodily competition and almost a full year in rehab to reach a 100% success status, physically. My mind didn't initially seem tarnished, but I think that was because I was too young to understand it all. Plus, it was like my brain erased it. Don't get me wrong, my disposition had shifted. What had defined me as being important was no longer available. I wasn't the superstar athlete in school anymore. I wasn't the pretty popular girl who hung out at Stud Row anymore. And I wasn't deemed a college prospect anymore. I had lost my starting positions to girls that I had competed with throughout the previous years, I no longer had friends, I got down to almost eighty-five pounds, and I had fake bonded teeth that would occasionally fall out. I had all the reasons to back away from the spotlight, and that's what I began to do.

Luckily, by the last quarter of my sophomore year, the doctors gave me clearance to play sports. At that time in the semester, it was softball season. I knew I could regain some level of my popularity by getting back on the playing field. I had been one of the leaders of that team at 14 years of age and a 100 pounds of talent. Maybe I still had that superpower. Fortunately, during pre-scheduled training, I was able to regain some of my focus as well as full extension of my right arm. On the other hand, the outlook of the rest of my life had become a bit of a dark cloud. Sports had protected me from getting jumped at school. Without them, the doors would open back up to more bullying. I wouldn't know the psychological ramifications that my car wreck would have on me until I was in my late thirties.

As I processed that short-lived era, I realized that I had been completely absent from Rudy. Who took care of him that entire time? Where was he in all of it? How did he make it through the rehab sessions, doctor visits, and summer school classes that I ended up having to take after my dad discovered how many days I ditched? I was in ICU, so he had to pull me out of school two weeks early. Nobody knew if I was going to live or not, and then he had to find out how dishonest I had been. What a disappointment I was for taking advantage of his trust.

Even more disturbing was that I didn't even remember the significance of my dog enough to make sure if he was being fed. I may have entered into a period of hidden low self-esteem and uncertainty, but that was no excuse. He didn't ask to be neglected. I understand that shit happens in life and we deal with it how we do. But as I look back today, who was there for my Rudy? Who was there to keep him nourished and hydrated? Who was there to play with him and give him the exercise he needed? Who was there to share love and cuddles with him, and show him how much he meant to us? It was my Pops... the one who was always there for my dogs. How blessed was I to have a dad who made sure Rudy was alright? If I could go back in time, I'd remember my dog more. I'd remember his essence. I'd remember that he, too, needed healing and reassurance. So much for shifting my modality on my priorities.

I was almost 16 years old and, shortly thereafter, both of my parents had merged into new relationships. My mom's partner was closer to her in age and had a super cool vibe and personality. He treated me great and, in no time, even him and my dad became best friends. Back then, nobody could fathom divorcees getting along, much less them and their new significant others. I remember some of my friends actually asking me if they were having 3-sums together. It was hilarious and the first of the amicable interactions between exes that I knew of. They totally made it work. They'd go fishing together, take trips to Denver, attend all of my games and events together, drank beer together, worked on projects together, cooked dinners, and had deep mentoring conversations. How lucky of a kid was I not to have to grow up with such angry parents or any type of division?

I didn't know how they did it. But, because they put bygones aside and made me and my future their priority, we were able to live as a happy combined family. The way they chose to handle the breakup of their loving connection showed me that just because things don't turn out as planned, doesn't mean they can't turn into something wonderful. I must've stored that sense of perception somewhere, because it would help me enjoy a few of my relationships and both sides of exes later on in my adult years.

While my three amigos were paving the road for me to travel on to my next level of teenagerhood, my dad also became pretty serious with his new lady friend. The only problem was that her energy wasn't close to the easy-going type of frequency as my mom's new boyfriend. I think it had more to do with me than with her though. She never treated me badly. I just didn't feel that she was genuine. It didn't seem like she really loved my dad. I'm not sure if that was the beginning of the intuitive gifts I would get in my gut, or if I was just being a selfish brat. Within a few months of her and my dad dating, they decided to move into a new home together. I was instantly pissed, jealous, and began acting like I had no rules or boundaries. I didn't know what it was about her that I couldn't connect with, but I wasn't having it. I was certainly not about to share a living space with her. I felt like she was taking my dad away from me, so I was angry.

How dare me not take into consideration my dad's feelings and what made him happy. How dare me make things so difficult for a parent that did everything for me. Yet, that was my reality and the type of teenager I had become from that interaction. There wasn't anything that could justify my behavior other than me learning the hard knocks for myself. When they showed me the new room and bathroom that I'd be sharing with her daughter, I walked out the door without saying a word, and sat in my dad's truck pouting. At that very second, I decided to go live with my mom. I must've been stuck in the dustiest cloud of my life because that meant giving up my dog. Rudy was the love of my life, my best friend, my everything. But my mom's 2-bedroom ground-level detached apartment had no yard, and did not permit pets. Therefore, my insensitive ass would leave Rudy behind for good. I was his human and I abandoned him.

I didn't give my dad's new relationship or home any more thought than I had to. I didn't even take into account that they didn't have a yard for Rudy either. For the next year, my poor little Pomeranian remained tied to a tree while anxiously waiting for me to come visit. In the beginning, I was there every day. But as I approached my Sweet Sixteenth, I became too busy. He had been a part of my life for over eight years, and I was too occupied with senseless stuff to stop by and give him a miniscule of the love and attention that he longed for. If I did make time, I'd see his helpless self bound to the trunk exasperated from being so excited to see me. Another "how dare me," right? How dare me not make him my number one. How dare me just give him up and not have the decency to make it work? Age wasn't just a number and, in no way, could be blamed for that type of cruelty. I knew better and was taught better. Trust that I've paid a lifelong price carrying around that horrendous guilt ever since.

My dad gave Rudy all the love he could while trying to juggle his new relationship and coparenting duties with my mom. He came to the conclusion that Rudy deserved more. He deserved more time, attention, friendship, presentness, and more everything. My dad had given me one last chance, and I didn't pull through. That following 9th year of having Rudy, he gave him away. He had done his research and found a wonderful, and extremely fitting, home with an older woman who couldn't wait to share her life with a furry companion and best friend. He never officially told me. I went to visit one Sunday afternoon and Rudy wasn't there. That exit would be my second assignment and one of my harshest with the concept of completion.

My dad's relationship didn't last much longer after Rudy had been gone, and he moved into a place of his own. He never really settled down again seriously with another woman. He dated around and had his well-deserved fun, but never needed anybody to fill his time. He was a lifelong musician, coach, fisherman, pool player, great friend, mentor, wise soul, intellect, great cook, and one of the most understanding people you'd ever meet. He taught me not to wait for anybody to make me happy because I'd always be waiting. My mom's boyfriend became my new stepdad, and those three would continue their travels and companionship to the fullest.

For me, I had already built up a good deal of sadness in my system. I went on with my ways, but always thought about what I did to my dog. It didn't help that our town was small and you couldn't fully get away from anyone. The wretched hole in my heart would expand anytime I'd be near the street where my dad used to live with him. I just never said anything about it. I stored the lesion somewhere in my body and adjusted to life with that deplorable pain.

Today, it would be ironic that my experience with Rudy would be one of the things I despise the most in families with pets, and the reason they get them in the first place. I cannot fault kids for being kids or teenagers for being teenagers. But I can fault parents who know better, and those who keep getting their kids pets when they're not being taken care of. Along with the ghastly upregulation of breeding, this is why there's such a problem with overcrowded shelters and homeless animals all over the globe. Animals are getting euthanized daily because so.

Bless my dad for trying, and for giving me the opportunity to learn from my own mistakes. He provided me with a fortune of love over and over again and I failed over and over again. Thank goodness he had the decency and respect for animals to take it upon himself and go align my dogs with better homes. He never gave them up to a shelter. He never surrendered them. He never abandoned them. Through it all, he too, finally learned a lesson.

2
The Solar Plexus: Doing – Being – Identifying

I entered young adulthood without a pet and the accommodating responsibility. I wish I could say that I was coming into my age with a clean slate, but I had already begun to repress built-up shame and guilt for the mistakes I made in my youth. It didn't stop me from attending two colleges, traveling around the country to watch pro-baseball games, venturing to New York for a modeling gig, and then landing in Los Angeles for the next twenty years striving to be rich and famous. I was out in the world, on my own, hustling, and trying to find my way. I was mingling with celebrities, inundated in the illusion of the industry, and caught up in the hype of the money and influential platform it could someday provide for me and my family. As I explored life's avenues, jobs, relationships, and spiritual wellness, I found myself on everyone else's time and schedules. Luckily, I was mature enough by then, and had acquired a significant amount of mindfulness, not to bring an animal into my home. I already had so many obligations that I just didn't want to neglect another pet.

I did, however, have a live-in companion and best friend in the form of a laminated smiley face cut out from a plastic tablecloth and glued to a popsicle stick. His name was "Spiffy" and he went everywhere with me, and I mean everywhere. I had created him after working a few days as one of the lead actresses on a movie set. It shot during graveyard hours and almost seventy-five miles outside of the city in a town called Lancaster. Someone had slacked on the production team and hadn't arranged hotel rooms for the crew. For the first three or four days, us spoiled actors had to drive ourselves back and forth to the location until our suites became available. The only problem was that, by the time shooting wrapped every morning, it was 6am and at the peak of rush hour traffic.

Anybody who knows about the transportation in LA could affirm that our commute was like driving through a gridlock of hell. Going ten miles at certain times of the day could take most of the afternoon. Try working on a set for twelve hours, being exhausted, and having to drive back home bumper to bumper with road ragers honking their horns and flipping their fingers. I decided that instead of circulating that energy, I'd give people something to smile about, and literally. That's when Spiffy came into my life and changed everything. I made five other similar emoticons of Spiffy's cousins and distributed them to the other leading cast members. I knew the powerful and uplifting influence he had on all those that came into contact with him while he was with me. So, it wasn't a surprise when I'd hear similar stories from the other actors throughout my time there. He was my road dog. He was my soulmate. He was my everything. And for the rest of my stay in that city, he would be what kept me going.

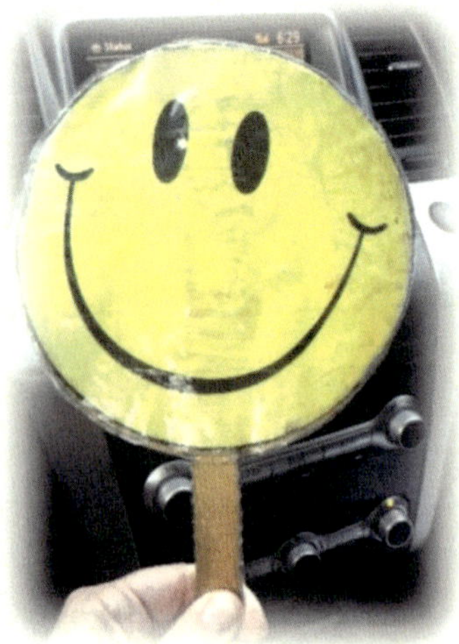

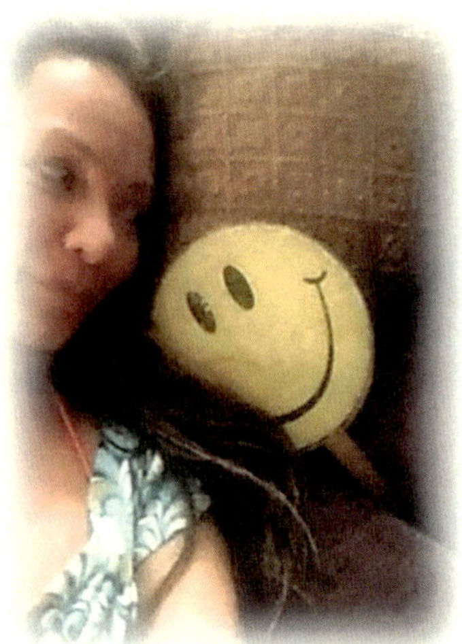

Everybody from back home had told me how difficult it would be to make it in Tinseltown. Yet, it happened for me almost overnight. I lived in trendy West Hollywood, had a lucrative paying cocktail job in the VIP room of one of the hottest venues in the city, was in a top acting class, went to a prime gym, and was booking commercials and films. Then, just like that, my dad died. The true love of my life, my best friend, my everything, suddenly passed away of a heart attack.

I was in complete shock and so were my mom and stepdad. He seemed just fine twenty-four hours earlier. We spoke every day on the phone and I was planning on bringing him up to live with me in the next couple of months. To make matters worse, he had called me the night before and I was too tired to pick up. I had been working extra shifts and figured that I'd call him back later after getting some rest. He left a message telling me that he was at my mom and stepdad's eating tortillas and watching the Lakers game like they always used to do together. Then he followed with how much he loved me. I never heard his voice again.

In the midst of my starlit dreams, I was now fighting for air. I went from shock to anger to guilt to sadness to fear; sometimes in order, sometimes mixed in with each other. I'd go to work every Friday and Saturday night and put on my happy mask in that power environment like everything was alright. I'd go on auditions and hide the pain that I was feeling. I even took an offer to leave my amazing cocktail job to take what I thought would be an even more amazing, flexible, and financially secure job. And instead, I lost both jobs. My income began depleting and my talent reps dropped me. Add to that, wrecking my car and having to abruptly move out of my apartment. All of this was going on while also getting sabotaged by competitive girls and duped by unfaithful dudes. The last bit of strength and will I had left didn't seem to be enough to carry me through.

I became numb to everything and quickly spiraled into depression. I never told anyone, not even my parents. Yet, after somewhat recovering, how in the world didn't people know? I saw pictures and I was skin and bones. It would take me three years before I could fully peel myself off my empty floor. I was living with barely any furniture for the first five months of that period. I would sit there and cry for ten hours a day as everything was falling apart. I didn't think things could get any worse after death, but they did. Somehow, I kept going. After looking back, it says a lot when you can overcome and conquer so much sadness and defeat all alone, and still go on.

Thank goodness I continued reading and writing. I wrote in my journals, I wrote poetry, scripts, and I read and wrote books. I went to acupuncture weekly for two years and felt major improvements. It was the best credit card debt I had ever accrued. Days got better and then, some days, they'd feel worse than they'd ever been. On those good days, I'd take advantage and go to the gym. That was my only means of social activity. Yet, I'd be lucky if I could make the entire drive without pulling off into some parking lot to bawl my eyes out.

I eventually became a robot. I told myself that I'd never again go through that much pain and hurt like that in my heart. By 2005, I'd be tested once more, as I lost my best friend from back home. And although guilt tried to creep in for making the same type of selfish decision the last time I spoke to him, as I did with my dad, I didn't let it. By that time, I had already developed a steel-coated chest plate, which allowed me to view his passing much differently.

I was sad that I didn't have him in physical form anymore, and just as sad for shafting him the last time I ever spoke to him. He had driven into town from college to see me one Christmas when I was back home visiting. I blew him off and met up with an ex-boyfriend from college instead. The next morning, he was pissed at how inconsiderate I was for leaving him hanging. Thinking that he'd get over it, as we had spent twelve other wonderful years enjoying much happier moments, I didn't pay any attention to it. I knew he headed back to the southern part of the state that day, because he sent me an email later on from campus reminding me how insensitive I was to pull the stunt that I did. I was going to sit on it for a few days before responding, but he died that week. Not only didn't I get to say goodbye, but I didn't get the chance to say that I was sorry. What a thoughtless asshole I was to choose a one-night fling over one of my most precious soul connections.

I took the guilt bullets and lodged them up into my body parts underneath my armor. Unbeknownst to me which ones, I continued to soldier on. I ended up spending almost twenty years in Hollywood chasing a dream that gradually became unfulfilling. I went out there with an abundance of creativity, authenticity, and fearlessness, not to mention some decent looks and an outgoing personality. And for a short time, I was slightly rewarded for it all. But the typecasting, power tripping, backstabbing, cheating, and extreme levels of sexism were staggering. Plus, who you knew seemed to be vital in making you or breaking you. As for relationships, I never needed one to make things better. Yet, it would've been nice to meet a good guy. Plenty of seekers showed up, and I had my fair share of celeb and athlete hookups. But there was rarely any genuine significance for anything to last more than a few months.

I'm sure it didn't help that I didn't kiss people's asses and had my own beliefs and opinions, as well as my perception of originality. That didn't sit well with many, especially my acting coaches and certain agents. It would be an ongoing battle just trying to be who I was, and like who I was. For most of my participation in that business, wearing a bikini and sexy tight clothing was my identity. It didn't matter how classy I represented myself, or how separated I kept from the nightlife scene. Nor, did the time I dedicated to studying, crafting my skills, and the spiritual aspects of my soul make any difference. I was still placed into a category void of talent and substance. It was unbelievable how many people told me that I'd never make it. I guess I couldn't blame anyone for not taking an interest in me for substantial projects. I had filmed several commercials, but my film and television works were weak. Not to take away from anyone else's involvement, results, and content. But at that time in my life, that was what I dealt with.

I remained determined and persistent that I would prove everybody wrong. I did all I could to keep focused on my visions and goals so that I wouldn't be labeled a failure. I actually thought I could change Hollywood for the better. What in the galaxy was I thinking? Then, after years of being exposed to toxic mold, dealing with over a hundred symptoms, and getting scammed out of thousands of dollars from the attorney representing me in that health matter, I was forced to take a seat and reevaluate my direction. LA and the accumulation of the entertainment business were not benefiting me both personally or professionally. And now, it was affecting me physically and emotionally. I had changed theatrical reps, genres, residences, and completed four remarkable seasons as a co-host on a game show. Yet, that energy hadn't been anywhere opulent since the first few years I was out there. The handful of wonderful people and auditions, the food, culture, crystal shops, diversity, the beautiful palm trees, the ocean, and the sunny moist weather were what kept me there.

I still hung on and stayed positive regardless of the uncertainty. But by 2014, two of my most cherished and respected agents had died within months of each other. Some inspiring actors and directors had passed, and one of my favorite fashion designers had kicked the bucket. All those dreams of working on projects under the direction of some of the greatest, while attending the premieres in one of his dresses, all went to pieces. I felt my aspirations slipping away and hope becoming a missed opportunity.

From then on, it seemed as if I was just going through the motions and acting like it was working out. Yet, the more I chased that dream, the farther it went. The harder I worked, the harder it got. The more I tried to let go and let it work itself out, the more it didn't work out. Then, in 2015, I tore my PCL playing basketball. Four months later, both of my thumbs began repeatedly breaking on the court as well. The one area that kept me happy was taken away from me. Why was I always losing and struggling? I felt like so much of my time out there was spent keeping my head above water. I had undoubtedly lost my air when my dad died in 2000. But why couldn't I get it back?

I went to numerous healers during my course out there to help me forgive myself for not picking up the phone that day. I thought I had addressed that issue to the deepest part of my component, but that guilt never left my system. For over seventeen years, I just couldn't let go of that decision. I always wondered if it had something to do with why the majority of LA wasn't working for me. Actually, why everything seemingly didn't work for me... since the day my dad died.

I remember receiving a message from the Universe late in 2016 when one of my upstairs neighbors was moving out. She was originally from gorgeous San Diego and had lived in my same Beverly Hills apartment complex for several years. She was such a kind-hearted being who dedicated herself to non-profit work for the betterment of surrounding communities. I wanted to say my goodbyes that last week before she moved back but, surprisingly, she was relocating to Tennessee. It was quite a shock. I asked her why such a drastic change since the weather was so nice where we were at. She replied, "Yes, the weather is. But the people aren't." That statement would never leave my mental apparatus again.

About six months later, I was completing the final touches on one of my published books when I spilled my protein shake on my keyboard. The plan was to turn in the manuscript that morning, so I was beside myself that my laptop stopped working. I immediately called all over town to see who could help. But to my dismay, nobody felt it was worth trying to save. Finally, I came across a computer tech in Glendale that felt he could revive it. I rushed out the door and found that my truck had been broken into. What in the world was going on? First my computer, now this. The two months of clothes and toiletries I had gathered for the homeless at the Los Angeles Mission and Women's Shelter had been stolen. I didn't think anything of it when I loaded the goods into my vehicle the night before with plans to deliver that next afternoon. Everything was swiped, including my basketballs and tennis racquets.

I raced down to my neighborhood gym to see if anyone tried to sell the sporting gear at discount. But I was out of luck. Nobody showed up. The panic dug into my Solar Plexus, so I sat in my vehicle for a minute to wipe away my armpit sweat and calm my meridians. When I dried off, and felt a bit more sensible, I pulled out from the street parking space. Then, CRASH!!! A car swerved to the inside lane and wrecked into the left side of mine. I was there turning in a report and talking to witnesses for a few hours. Then I managed to drive my mangled SUV home. I never got to Glendale, and didn't make my book deadline. My truck was in the shop for the next couple of weeks. I guess I was being sent another message to slow down and be patient.

Shortly thereafter, light signals were installed at the corner of our safe, quiet street and a new apartment complex began to go up across from my unit. That meant a ton of gardeners and construction workers casing the area. I never had a problem with security in any of my residences the entire time I lived in LA. Within days of the changes, my house got broken into and my shady landlord brought a city inspector inside my apartment while I was taking a shower. I'd been having tenant issues with him for quite some time, but that was the final straw. If all the signs during my entire tenure in that city weren't enough to heed caution, then the recently dangerous energy surrounding my living area would be my final warning to get out.

3
The Sacral Heart: Connecting With Something Beautiful From Something Awful

One afternoon in early June, I came into contact with someone I faintly knew during my teens. I was familiar with him and his family, but only because I went to school, and played sports, with his younger sibling. I found it odd that someone I never had any interaction with would suddenly pop up on my messenger asking me to dinner. He thought I lived in Scottsdale, and was there visiting. I wasn't interested, but decided to stay in communication platonically. That choice would be the catalyst to a seemingly blossoming partnership.

After a month and a half of talking on a daily basis via text and phone, he persuaded me into taking a trip back to my hometown to visit and spend time with my parents. When I got there, it hit me like a brick: I was back in a culture, lifestyle, and energy field that I had left almost two decades earlier. The place was filled with crime, corrupt politicians, haters, cheaters, stodginess, and alcoholics to say the least. The scenery looked like it hadn't changed a bit, and one inhale of that dry, hot, desert air brought back all the stale memories. I tried to maintain an open mind, but a rock instantly wedged itself in the pit of my stomach and never went away the entire time I stayed.

My new friend was approaching his 50's, recently divorced, and shared custody of two high school boys. Most of the guys I dated didn't have kids, and only one had been previously married. Maybe it was because LA was filled with youthful energy and I had attracted younger men. I never saw myself as being an older stepmom, much less a stepmom. He ran his own company and had zero affiliation with showbiz. In no time, I got a taste of his other interests. He chauffeured me to some of his hot spots that included an upscale gym, the bars he rotated through, and some of the top eateries. It seemed like he was a big shot and had quite a bit of pool around the city.

I wasn't physically attracted to him, but his personality, charm, and sense of humor began to shift me. We shared many of the same non-political views and non-religious beliefs, and seemed to click on quite a few topics. He appeared extremely kind-hearted, but I had a feeling that he was the type of guy who probably got taken advantage of. He seemed to be well put together and financially grounded in the upper middle class. But from his stories, people targeted him like vultures. I knew he had a deep love for his sons from all of our talks, so something told me that they gave him the strength to shrug it off.

One week turned into two weeks and on to four. He wined and dined me, took me shopping, catch-and-release fishing, drove me to see my parents, and threw barbecues for me to meet his and the rest of his large family. He also treated me to a haircut and massage from one of the deluxe salons. He seemed enamored with my writing and spiritual work, but couldn't stop lathering me with compliments for what I had achieved as an actress. Everyone he brought around was calling me a movie star. I could tell that I was back in a small town because I was nowhere close to being a movie star. I wished that I had a list of films we could stream, but I was a no-name in Hollywood. It was flattering to see how high of a pedestal people put me on.

When I was finally ready to return to LA, he asked me to come back and stay for good. I thought he was out of his mind. No matter how dispassionate the scene had become for me, I'd never leave Los Angeles. I was frustrated with that city and all the stress it had caused me, but it was all I had known for almost half of my life. I had spent my blood, sweat, tears, and oxygen developing what I thought was a network of business associates and friendships. I lived in my own apartment, on my own schedule, and had my own formulas for what kind of food and supplements I put in my body. I had a workout regimen, played basketball, wrote books, poetry, and scripts, held energy and stretching sessions, meditated, and watched my top shows on tv. I had earned my independence and honed in on it to the fullest. I couldn't move backwards and relocate to a state that I eagerly wanted out of. I couldn't give everything up to be a stepmom and work in a business I had no knowledge of. I had been in a slump, but I was still ambitious. I had a lot on my plate to accomplish.

His excitement and enthusiasm were so impressive that he had me contemplating whether or not I should make the move. He had such a playful attitude that I knew he'd be a lot of fun. Then he threw out the ideas of starting up our own businesses and doing what we truly loved, so that we could live the best lives for the rest of our lives. We discussed keeping my place in LA, my friends, my aspirations, and being able to continue working in the acting profession. Plus, I'd be closer to my parents. Before I knew it, I was back in Los Angeles packing up what I could fit into my SUV.

People were puzzled that I was making such a sporadic move with someone I barely knew. Yet, I felt like the encounter and opportunity came to me at the time it did for a reason. I had never looked for love, was never desperate for love, or ever needed to be in a relationship to feel loved. Honestly, guys had been nothing but stomach aches and distractions for me. Yet, he seemed like such a great guy. Maybe I was coming into the companionship that I felt I always deserved. Maybe the Universe was telling me to take a chance and get out of my comfort zone; to explore other options and other types. Maybe it was good karma coming to pay me back for all the amazing things I had done for others in my 43 years of existence. I thought about how I made the best of things and kept going all those years after being defeated. I had always followed the rules, bought all the books, took all the classes, did what I was told, and never stepped on anyone. I had unquestionably paid my dues. I just wondered if the cyclic nature of good energy was finally coming back to bless me.

Before making the sixteen-hour drive, we spent the last few days living it up in Los Angeles. I was excited to share with him some of the things that I still loved about that city. We went to a few of my favorite places to eat, hit up the Laugh Factory, shopped, and spent time at the beach. We also drove through the Hollywood lights and slums, so that he could get a better idea of LA's uniqueness other than what the antagonists, news stations, and gossip sites had portrayed it to be. Right before we left, I arranged for my wonderful neighbors to housesit my place since I was reassured that I could go back every month, whenever I wanted, and/or any time I had to work.

It took a couple of days to unpack and get acclimated to his home. Everything seemed okay, but I couldn't shake the precarious feeling in my pancreas. There was something in my gut that kept telling me that things weren't right. I continued to remind myself that change was scary and it would just take some time. I had already begun energy coaching as a side job, so I had learned years of techniques and methods to undermine and disable fear and stress. I was a huge advocate of meditation among a plethora of natural remedies for maintaining a healthy mind-body-spirit balance. When my partner suggested that we remodel the bottom guest room into a Zen room, I was ecstatic!

I had accumulated an array of crystals, Buddha statues, art, symbols, animals, books, candles, pictures, and spiritually hippy décor throughout the years. Since developing quite a knack for designing on a budget, I felt like my places of residence were eccentrically tailored to my energy and beliefs. I always dreamed of having an extra room designated as sacred. Now, I was getting my own personal space to meditate, read, journal, study, pull oracle cards, EFT tap, conduct my energy sessions, or to simply sit in silence. All of my totems would finally have an area of indoor forest, land, ocean, sun, moon, and sky where they could be together, and with Spiffy.

My new temple had me feeling like maybe things were starting to come together, especially since it would give one of my fondest figures a place to call his own. I had recently brought one of my primary spirit animals back into my life. But because he was so large, I didn't have a comfy seat for him in my apartment. His name was "Bear" and it was unfair to him because I couldn't take him in the car with me like I did Spiffy. I couldn't just sit him on my bookshelf with my Tree of Life or Feng Shui fountains, or stick him in my gym bag to run errands. Since moving, I would have a new palace where he would fit in perfectly.

I had met him the last day I was in town visiting my parents for my 43rd birthday. My mom wanted to send me back to LA with something special, so she took me to a thrift store for an unexpected surprise. Once I walked in, my eyes went right to him. He had found me! We hadn't seen each other since May 14th of 1989 when my vehicle collided with his peripheral. A part of both of us died that day, but a part of both of us also rebirthed into something better. He was sitting in a chair waiting for me to walk over. As I got up close, the grounding force in his eyes softened and he said to me, *"I am sorry for hurting you."*

I cupped his cushy face with my hands and said, "You didn't hurt me, my dear. You helped me."

From that moment on, we never separated again. I had no doubt that Bear would be the tranquil spirit of that room. Not only would he gift the premise with healing powers, strength, and grounding forces to keep us rooted, but he'd also help emphasize the importance of quiet time, solitude, and rest. It would be just what I needed.

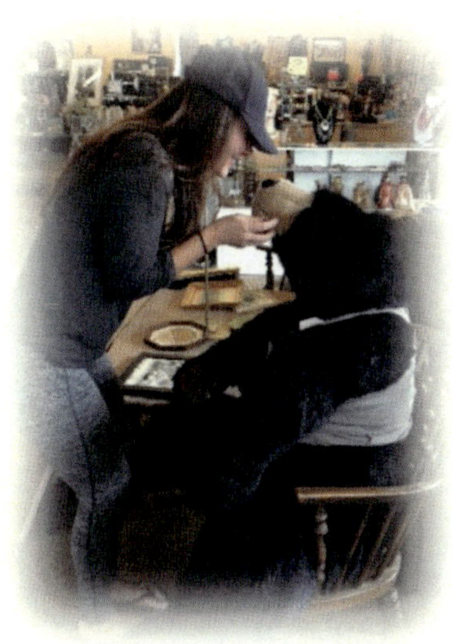

If I didn't think things could get any better, then I'd have think again. Within days of my arrival, I came into two life-changing connections in the forms of whiskers, paws, and furry anatomies. Each of my partner's sons had a dog of their own and they would bring them to our house after leaving the specified time with their mother. Instantly, we gravitated towards each other. Our energies were immediately interlinked. It was something so surreal; something so special. It was as if I was a little girl again meeting my new best friends. I introduced myself with a smile and an ear rub, and they reciprocated with the names: "Charly" and "Tippet!"

Charly was an 11-year creamy blonde purebred Chihuahua with beautiful eyes, lavish style, and a spring to her step. Tippet was a salt & peppered handsome 9-year mixed breed that my partner adopted for his younger son. They both had been brought into the previous home as puppies. I could tell that the dogs exuded quite a connective zest. They were vivacious as ever and each had specific identities and personalities. They definitely ran the show.

I hadn't had a pup since I was 16 years of age and, surprisingly, I wasn't a bit nervous. The encounter felt like it was happening accordingly and in my highest light. I knew the concept as "Divine Order" and had been something I explored throughout my metaphysical studies. I understood it as a way of embracing the aspect of perfect timing, and the power of the perception we choose to take when the illusion brings failure and pain. The only thing was that I detected some carelessness. I couldn't pinpoint it. But it brought me back to when I was those boys' same age, also unintentionally neglecting in my own way.

I didn't have to know much about the youngsters to see how spoiled they were by their father. I couldn't believe how they spoke to him and the fits that got thrown for the smallest things. The younger son seemed softer in nature, with an outgoing personality, and fairly friendly. Like many teenage boys, he had a room he couldn't keep clean where he stayed in bed much of the day playing video games. It appeared that self-sufficiency was non-existent in his world. I'd later learn that his dad didn't require him to do anything, and always picked up after him. Maybe that was because his mom enforced discipline. However, I did notice that he had a special closeness with Tippet. He actually had a fond love for both dogs.

With the older son, he also had no limitations. But there was something unpleasant in his demeanor and expressions. He reminded me of a horse fly trying to carry an identity of a butterfly. I couldn't pick up any genuineness from him, and I was pretty good at reading people from the start. I could've been wrong, but he seemed like a fake, resentful kid who was combative in the conformation of anything. I felt sorry for him because I could see his internal misery. I also knew that his energy was some type of warning.

To witness that kind of behavior so early on was unnerving. I tried to find some rationale to it, but all I could come up with was that we weren't raised the same. Therefore, we had different outlooks. Like many kids of that generation, they couldn't focus on anything other than their phones. Yet, studies were the basis for the younger son, and it showed. He was almost a straight-A student while also excelling in sports. When unglued, both boys enjoyed cool activities like football games, debate teams, and dating. I guess I could understand why full-time doggy care wasn't on their radar. Unfortunately, some veterinarian told them that it was healthy to crate the dogs for long periods. From the way I gathered it, on the weeks the boys spent at their mother's, Charly and Tippet stayed boarded the majority of the day, while she worked and they went to school (and played).

I hadn't had a dog for almost thirty years, but felt that I had become somewhat of an indirect animal activist. I had decreased my intake of meat throughout my stay in LA and disconnected from all wildlife captivation, which included zoos and marine parks that I loved so much as a child. I was against the usage of animals for medicine, entertainment, soups, rugs, and fashion, and strongly spurned the cruel practices of farmers. I detested puppy mills, backyard breeding, horse racing, rodeos, deforestation, and the callous inhumanity of shark finning. It was heartbreaking to walk into a pet store and see the display shelves of Betta fish stuck in little cups. Then I'd walk to the back and see the kitties and puppies caged up. I couldn't even stand to watch animals eating other animals on wildlife television shows. I had followed rescues and kept up as much as I could with volunteer adoption events in Los Angeles, and I had never heard that it was healthy to crate a dog for that long. It was appalling. Why would anyone have a pet if they were going to put them in a cage all day?

I don't think any vet would appreciate being confined in a closet for hours without the privilege of playtime, meals, fresh air, or a separate space to use the toilet. Certainly, they wouldn't be happy about having to sit in their own piss and shit for any length of time. It doesn't take being a doctor to know the benefits of exercise. No animal should be in a locked box so that their bodies can cramp up and bones stiffen, as well as lose their sanity and brain function.

I remember that instance as being the spark in changing the course of my career. It also opened my eyes as to what kind of people I was dealing with. My partner and his ex-wife seemed like decent people, but they probably shouldn't have owned pets. In a way, I could understand where the kids were coming from. They were teenagers absorbing a globe of information. I didn't like it, but I knew I was once there myself to some degree. From that moment until the chapter closed on the partnership, I treated those boys with extreme kindness as if they were my own. I just gave thanks that they weren't, and went on creating a loving family atmosphere as best as I could.

The older son would eventually drop out of school within months of me living there, and the disregard of his dog, Charly, became more apparent. He was bunking at his friend's dorm on the college campus with free reign to do what he wanted. Come to find out, Charly had been left in a crate for so long, and not tended to, that she'd have to sit in her pee for hours. When he would bring her with him to get money from his dad, she looked increasingly worse. She smelled like urine, was extremely skinny, and had some trouble breathing. I guess the teen became too busy with other things.

We found ourselves dog sitting her quite often. I would take her to McDonald's for a plain patty and, after scarfing it down, she'd try to eat the carboard box. To see a little dog in that kind of position was tough, but I began using it as the perfect ploy to eventually have her living with us permanently. The visits began with us watching her for an afternoon, which led to a weekend and, finally, to the entire time.

As for Tippet, that was another story. He appeared to have bouts with anxiety. He had also been crated for the majority of the day. And likely because of no walks, exercise, or social interaction, he would chew through his paws, nails, carpet, and the cushions on his doggy bed. He'd run circles chasing air, bark at spirits and ghosts, and was also very skinny. They told me he was always that thin and weird, but I knew there was more to it. Tippet was unique; there was nothing weird about him. I could tell something had been holding him back from being able to fully express who he was. It reminded me of the same shield I wore when I tried to hide my vulnerability and emotions over my dad dying.

Both dogs had no indoor potty training and were fed processed kibble. My partner told me how upset he'd get with them pissing all over the carpet at the previous home. Aside from all the commotion, they were happy dogs. Yet, he still had issues with them. I begged him to let me take over and be their full-time pet mom, because I knew I had the power to make things better for everyone. That became my primary goal. I just had no idea the blessings that those 4-pawed beings would give me along that journey.

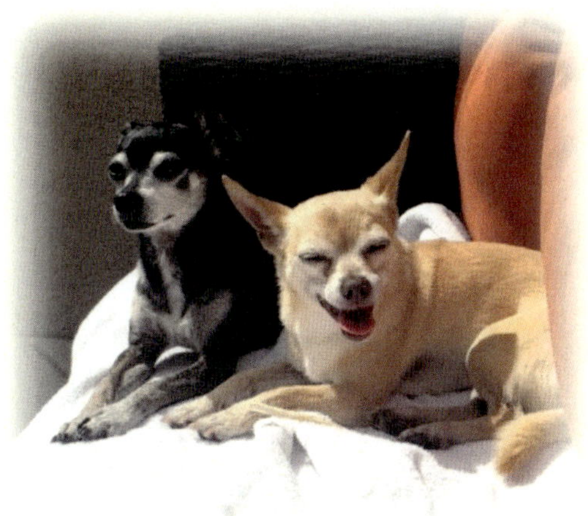

Within a month, both fur kids were with us permanently. When I wasn't driving around town with my partner giving estimates, I'd be home creating flyers, sales pitches, and social media posts to bring in business. Throughout the day, I'd work with them to help balance their potty habits. Plus, there were no more crates! They were free to use their limbs all day! We switched out their dog food, gave them more nutritious treats, and began taking them on daily walks. It was so beautiful to watch them come out of their shells and progress the way they did. Those dogs were already 9 and 11 years of age. And in spite of my partner telling me that they couldn't be trained, they got better, healthier, and younger. They even learned to use a newly installed doggy door. I was also learning how to care for an animal again. The Universe was giving me another chance to make up for being a kid. There was no way I was going to screw it up this time.

Down the road, my partner's oldest son secretly purchased a Teacup Chihuahua. I was livid that he would own another animal after neglecting his previous, but who was I fooling? He was a dishonest kid who didn't care about anyone but himself. Plus, he had recently turned 18 years old, so his father had no jurisdiction on his decisions or actions. The tiny dog was adorable, and after meeting her, Charly was devastated. She was like, *"What did I do wrong?"* The human she stood by for eleven years had replaced her, and so easily.

Then, after dog sitting her a few times, Charly realized how ungrateful her ex-human was. Quickly, her energy shifted, and she'd growl at him because she no longer liked him. It was still heart-wrenching to feel her pain in the beginning. Yet, it turned out to be rewarding. Not only did it bring us closer together and merge our internal components, but it sparked the activation of her Sacral, Heart, and Crown chakras. I knew she had healing powers upon meeting her. But after being displaced from everything she'd ever known, those tools ignited tenfold. Aside from discovering her horniness, she comprised a curative warmth of empathy. We were so much alike in being able to care and sense so deeply. She was a special little girl with a tangerine flair like that of an orange lotus filled with enlightenment and supreme consciousness. From the bond we had already developed, I knew that we'd be together forever.

As my elation for the dogs grew, so did the tension in the relationship. They became my priorities, so that meant taking time away from my partner and keeping us from doing the stuff he wanted to do. Like with kids, we had to take precautions to make sure nothing happened to them when we were away. We would have to leave lights on, make sure they had enough food and water, keep cords and electrical units out of reach, and come home at certain times to check on them. We couldn't travel anywhere that would keep us longer than twenty-four hours, because we couldn't leave them home alone. They weren't the type of pets that could be left at doggy day care establishments. I grew so close to them that nothing was as important as being with them. Maybe that was because I felt the maternal part of my femininity needing to nurture them. Or maybe, it was because something inside was telling me that it was finally time to get it right.

4
The Blue Throat and Third Eye: Going With the Gut… or Against It

I was starting to recognize that I was with a man who needed caressing 24/7. He had spoken of his attachments in our initial text conversations, but I had no idea the seriousness behind those statements. So, I ignored them. Cut to a few months later, and I was seeing how all the attention had to be on him. Therefore, the more time I spent with the dogs, and the closer we got, the more irritated he got. From their hair being everywhere, to his allergies, to allowing them on the furniture, to giving them filtered water, to taking them in the car with us, he was annoyed. Yet, he'd flip the switch and give them baths like a doting father would. He was just playing the part though. He didn't love them. He was just tolerating them to please me. Eventually, it would come at a price.

Relocating to what I thought could be an amazing adventure was turning into something dreadful. He had already shown signs of jealousy in snippets, but the emphasis put on the dogs accelerated it. His true colors were quickly making their presence. He was possessive, begrudging, and a roller coaster of moods. He'd also make up absurd claims that I was texting guys all day, as well as having affairs with every male I knew. Yet, it was him doing everything he was accusing me of. Talk about a walking double standard.

It was obvious that he needed to be in control. That was his power tool. To achieve that, he had to maintain a fake image. Yet, no matter how hard he attempted to be different, he couldn't. The odor of his nature was unmistakable. Maybe that's why he'd smell so sour every time he'd sweat or work out. I'd advise him to tweak his diet and explain how beneficial it would be to take time working through his mind. He'd see it as derogatory and bark back that I was picking on him. He made it clear that he didn't need anyone to heal him.

He also didn't need anyone to help him do anything. In his mind, he was an expert at everything. Yet, he'd talk about how other people were "know-it-alls." The envy was visible. He would make judgments in order to feel better about doing the same things. If you corrected him in any way, or tried to show him how to do it properly, he'd take it as a personal attack. Then he'd give you direction based on reliving his high school accolades. When he still couldn't get it right, he'd retort with, "Sorry, not everyone is as perfect as you."

I wondered why he was such an angry person when he seemed pretty well off in life. Then I remembered that things weren't usually what they seemed. I hadn't been there for five months and my whole life was changing into his. Everything was about him. From his schedule, his job, kids, friends, family, problems, sex, and insecurities, he was more important. Add to that, needing to be coddled constantly. His codependency was frightfully suffocating.

I didn't know if to listen to my gut, or to see it as a test since it wasn't something I had experienced. I convinced myself into thinking that he was just really into me. I actually felt sorry for the guy. I could tell that he lacked self-love. And like many who had crossed my path, I thought I could help him on his. Healing was my specialty and I knew I could strengthen his Root chakra enough for him to feel a comfortable sense of security. What a dangerous thought process to trick my mind into believing, because what I didn't see was that those were the early stages of an emotionally abusive, toxic situation.

As with everything in my life, I made the best of it. Then one night, he popped the question. We had both agreed that marriage and a ring weren't important, so I knew he was up to something. I was never interested in that route. I didn't even know how much longer I could put up with him, much less spend the rest of my life with him. My stupid ass felt so pressured not to hurt his feelings, that I said, "Yes." It was one of the most displaced moments of my entire existence.

From then on, I became bound by a matrimonial leash. He questioned me about every notification on my phone, inspirational post, comment, and random articles written about me on the internet. I was interrogated about affirmations I wrote in my journal, any guy I knew, people I stayed in contact with, the celebrities I met, all the trips I ever took, and every awesome story of my childhood. He even probed me why my mom was texting. I found myself having to explain a lifetime of details daily. Then he began isolating me from anything that made me happy. It started with the dogs and his continuous insults of how I was becoming a "helicopter mom"... on to sarcastic remarks of how I'd be "parent of the year" if I had kids. Finally, it led to my friends, my parents, career, interests, and spiritual practices. Before I knew it, I was losing every sense of my being.

For the first year, I felt like I was still somewhat strong-minded enough, and physically intact, to do my best and brush off his shitty attitude and offensive comments. But I was gradually being removed from myself. I was methodically being molded. I was participating in family gatherings, attending parent meetings, football games, drag shows, la crosse tournaments, banquets, and so much more in full support. I worked daily in his company and exercised with him at a gym where I wasn't allowed to look at, or talk to, anybody. Then I had to put up with him slurring what a "fucken bitch" I was at the end of the day after downing too many martinis.

By a couple of months into the second year, I had almost completely lost my personal freedom. I had gone on a few local auditions, but was barely working at all with acting. We also hadn't gone back to LA in some time. There wasn't any point to; I was inundated in his agenda. There was no time for silence, reading, or space to act, write, or network. I got an opportunity to pen a script and, because attention was taken off of him, he made it miserable. He'd slam doors and throw tantrums, not knowing what to do with himself while I was completely deep in my project. The majority of the time I could write was in the late-night hours, at the kitchen island, while he slept. And usually, he stayed up as long as he could laying on the couch on full radar night watch.

I managed to meditate any chance I could, and even that decreased. I wasn't able to exercise or stretch on my own, talk to my parents more than a few times a week, keep in contact with anyone, or listen to my own music. If I didn't pick up his calls or instantly return his texts, he would be fuming. He monitored my social media posts and threw constant fits for not publicly announcing our relationship.

I had to ask myself if I was doing the right thing by staying. Did I really think he was a good man who treated me like I deserved to be treated? If my dad was alive, he would've despised him. That, in itself, should've answered my questions no matter how many times I heard that relationships took work. No thanks. I was perfectly fine being single and soaring free like an eagle. The only reason I was still there was because of Charly and Tippet. He knew it and it scorched him like an inferno. I just happened to be on the other end taking it in like a burn victim. They were all that mattered to me, so I was willing to sacrifice everything for them.

Char and Tip had become my best friends and soulmates... as all of my dogs did. I couldn't explain the feeling I'd get every time I saw them beam with excitement when I'd stroll in the door, or when they knew we were taking them for a walk, ride, or hike. They just had this awareness of completeness being with me. We'd sit out on the backyard porch and gaze into the sun. I'd rub their bellies and see them engulfed in trust. Then on days when they each felt a little feisty, I'd bring out *Little Duckie*. How they loved that toy!

Even though their beds were in our room and in front of our king size, they'd still come lay down next to my side. When I'd take a shower, they'd sit on my dirty clothes in front of the glass door. Then, when I'd get out, Charly would lick the water off my legs. If I had to leave the room for any reason, day or night, she would track my every footprint. I could tell that she just wanted to make sure I wasn't going to leave. She was my little girl. I knew she'd follow me until the end of time, as I would her. She was something special. I started to suspect that maybe she was a therapy dog. I already knew of the emotional capacity that kept her Sacral chakra activated, but it was clear that she was just as mighty in her Third Eye with that type of intuition.

Tippet had similar mannerisms, but in his own way. If he was outside and I was working inside, he'd peek his head through the doggy door just to make sure I was still there. Then he'd go back out and lay in the hot rays. He also just wanted to make sure that I was close to him. I could see that Tippers was a doer in his Solar Plexus, but his Heart chakra was most sensitive. No matter how much bark he had over bite, he was a skinny bundle of love who reveled in daily pampering. He was also a cotton ball underneath his Darth Vader covering. They were both aware of the awful vibe in that household and, yet, their Anahatas were fully open.

There was no doubt that Char and Tip had their own formulas independently as well as together. Tippet would run on three legs and kick up dirt after peeing on a tree. Whereas, Charly would roll around on wet grass coated with poop smell. She could sense a dirtbag a mile away and made sure to let them know they weren't welcome in our home. Tip could race and leap like a cheetah, and probably because his colossal sized ears acted as his antennas. The only problem was that he was a bit disconnected. I knew it had something to do with the anxiety he developed from all those years being crated. There would be times where he'd unknowingly walk out the front door. After frantically searching for him, we'd find him almost a mile away confusingly trying to cross the main street. His internal compass was definitely a work in progress, so we had to keep a close eye on him.

We didn't have concerns in that area with Charly because she appeared to be extremely cerebral. She just had to go at her own pace. On occasion, she'd get a sore front leg from too much walking or hiking. So, she had to ease up. Sometimes I'd carry her down the peak or ensuing path so she wouldn't be in discomfort. Just as we began thinking the limping was due to age and arthritis, she'd become a speedster at the park when she was off of her leash. Charly never ceased to amaze me. She wasn't lacking in the intelligence, limbic, or party girl categories. She would eat human treats until she passed out sitting upright and, other times, perform her trademark *Cha Cha Cha* dance while we scratched her butt.

Make no mistake... they did need their space and quiet time, especially when Tip would get into a few of his grouchy moods. Char would let him steal Duckie periodically and allow him to sit in her spot on my lap. She would keep distant and let him work out his issues. Yet, she always made it known that she was the boss no matter what she supposedly and temporarily gave up. She was the glue, the strength, and the foundation of that union. That's why they were so perfect for each other. I began seeing how distinct every single day was with them, and how being present was what made it so valuable.

I found it funny how they hated so many of my partner's friends, except his best friend. But they loved my parents. It was that old adage that dogs were the best judges of character. It just showed me the type of people that were in our surroundings. I knew the uniqueness of animals, but I became convinced that they were so much more. They were enlightened beings that would come to us in and out of our lives... depending on the direction we were headed and the tasks that needed to be completed. They were Totems that would teach us, inspire us, and bring us back to the center of our souls, our home, to help us remember our power and purpose.

I started catching on to how my partner would use them in order to manage me. He had already thrown me out several times, then lured me back in with, "I'm sorry, I won't do it again," and, "We've invested so much together." Yet, he couldn't evict the dogs. Even though his kids didn't spend any time taking responsibility for either of them, he'd still rub it in my face that they were always theirs and not mine. I realized that the dogs were his control tools. And, as long as he allowed them to be with me, he would have access to me.

I began to implement his own moves to benefit the three of us. I'd go along with his plans as long as it included Charly and Tippet. Before I knew it, they were traveling with us everywhere, especially to his son's sporting events. We'd only go to dog-friendly restaurants, sneak them into our hotel rooms and stadiums, and go out every few minutes to check on them. My plan was working out for everyone, because he got to be with me and I got to be with the dogs.

It was mid-year, and some days, it had me thinking that I could still make things work. Then I'd come back to my senses and realize that it was only getting worse. He was putting me down more than putting me on a pedestal. He was no longer intrigued with my past acting adventures, energy healing missions, and literary projects. In fact, he hated everything. And since the somewhat pretty ring he gave me hadn't fully succumb me yet, he was even more peeved. Fancy jewels had never been my means of worth or symbol of commitment. And I lived in Beverly Hills where extravagant bands were the norm. But when we'd be back visiting, fingers sported an average of four carats. I could've cared less, but the look on his face was always priceless.

Those kinds of instances would seed more polarity. One minute, he'd be buying copies of one of my published pieces to help promote me, and set up book-signing events. The next, he'd be telling me how disturbing it was to read about my sex life in Los Angeles and what a whore I was. That was coming from a guy who gawked at, and flirted with, huge-boobed females right in front of me. My book detailed situations, examples, and methods aimed at helping my readers along their own paths. It just so happened that a handful of them were related to sensuality; not mine personally. Plus, they were funny. So, it was obvious where his attention was drawn to and even more apparent how disgusted he was with himself. That was why he couldn't handle all the other pages filled with self-empowerment. He couldn't deal with people getting better. Unfortunately, most of those copies have been shelved ever since.

The layer of degradation was only one of many, as his insecurities were triggered regularly. His friends would ask how he got a girl like me, that I was too good for him, and settled for him. Those he didn't know thought I was his daughter. He'd be inflamed and I'd have to hear about it for days. If that wasn't hell, then all the times I'd appear on tv would be. He'd put me down for watching the game show I had worked on almost ten years earlier. He'd belittle my performance and tell me that I was "full of myself" and someone who just "needed attention." I don't know if he felt bad for the hurtful things he said, or if it was his way of keeping me from realizing my worth. But then he'd switch it up and act like he was kidding. The continuous mental compression actually had me believing what he said, hating what I looked like, and finding reasons to be angry at the production.

I was able to go back to LA a few times, but rarely without him. Plus, he'd always create something to fight about and ruin the entire stay. He even left me there once with no money or way to get back. Then he caught a return flight the next day with promises that he'd change. That broken record didn't last long, but it got me home. I thought I'd finally wake up, but before I could blink, I lost my apartment. My established self was decaying and my days were inching closer to not owning anything. Other than going back to take his son, and for a few health appointments, the trips to LA stopped.

As we approached the end of the year, every part of my system was on fire. Not only was my menses so uncomfortably irregular, but then I'd have to deal with being accused of faking them. Within six weeks of living there, my hair began falling out, I was sleep deprived, and had developed skin allergies, gas, and blurry vision. My ring finger also became sore and swollen. It was like my body was shielding me from wearing that finger cuff, as well as him touching me. I knew my internals were trying to tell me something. I also knew that it was causing my body to drastically change.

It was tough to digest that my looks were going south and I was prematurely aging overnight. Since it was like a world war going to the gym together, I hadn't worked out on a consistent basis for almost two years. My entire life was spent playing sports, exercising in a fitness center, or in some way, being active. From college throughout my entire employment in the LA workforce, I was mostly hired for jobs based on my physical appearance. I couldn't work out in public with him and only felt safest playing tennis on a faraway outdoor court in the daytime. That way I didn't have to be scolded for looking anywhere near another man, or have to deal with him wanting to thrash any guy focusing on me or my body. I had never been over 117 pounds in my life and I was pushing 141. I became so physically ugly that I lost my confidence, oomph, and ambition. I was incredibly self-critical and couldn't stand to look in the mirror. It made me stay home and away from people. From the talk around town, that was his perfect opportunity to cheat on me.

I didn't know how to find help, healing, or my way anymore. I for sure couldn't see a clear exit plan. My mom knew something was going on. But she didn't truly detect the seriousness of danger that was taking shape because my smile hid it. Honestly, I was embarrassed and ashamed to disclose any information to anyone, much less her. People had their own crap to deal with, why burden them with mine? I was so disappointed in myself for ending up in that position in the first place. How could I have ever allowed anyone to inhibit me, make me hate myself, kill my hope, and remove my light? I literally couldn't face my own face in the glass reflection. So, how could I face anybody else with that bullshit?

Meditation with myself and my spirit guides was my only form of communication and remedy I had left to keep me from losing my freaken mind. It was also slipping away. My partner wouldn't let me out of his sight or grips. When I did have a few minutes to sit in the Zen room and be in a space of calmness with the dogs, he would barge in and call me "selfish." He hated that I wouldn't reciprocate with anger, and that I could consciously remain in a domain of peace. Being that the dogs went in there to receive their higher vibrations as well, he'd continue to throw more insults.

Since he wasn't getting the responses he wanted, he decided to take matters in a different direction. Instead of picking on me, and at me, he started picking on Tippet. He would pretend to be interested in playing with him on the floor, or on the stairs, and quickly begin play fighting with him way too aggressively. Really, though, I could sense that he was instigating him to lose his temper.

He would forcibly roll Tippet back and forth to the point where Tip would start feeling threatened. I'd tell him not to be so rough and, every single time, he would respond with some complete nonsense that Tippet knew he was just playing. That was an absolute lie. There was nothing Tippet perceived as fun and playful during those interactions. My partner would get more intense with him to the point that Tippet had no choice but to defend himself. Therefore, he'd bite him. Instantly, my partner would throw Tippet on his back and constrain him with authority by digging his hand into his chest. He would get right into Tip's face with a scathing look, and chew him out. Without letting up, he'd then look over at me and tell me that Tippet had to submit and learn who the boss was.

A piece of my heart would get ripped out every time I saw him do that to Tippet. He was so confused. He didn't know how to play because he'd get punished for it. He'd be laying there, on his back, looking at me with fright in his eyes like, *"What did I do?"* No wonder he had the issues he had. When he was in my care, I couldn't love him and Charly enough. I gave them all of my attention and instilled trust and strength inside their furry little cores. I knew they both felt safe and protected, especially Tippet, by the way their physical, spiritual, mental, and emotional bodies elevated.

Charly was extremely confident and, although she battled with internal fears of being replaced again, self-esteem wasn't an area she needed work on. She danced to her own beat. In his own unique way, Tip moved mountains and flew just as freely. Yet, my partner was slowly crushing him like he was doing to me. He'd be nice to him one moment, and the next he'd bully and provoke him. He'd manipulate his little brain, his organs, and his perception. Being a nervous wreck was clearly a sign of how misled his poor little mind was. Tippet was pure innocence. He didn't deserve any of that. I couldn't ever figure out why, at times, he'd snap at Charly. From then on... I knew.

It was sad being around a miserable person who got his kicks off making a defenseless dog miserable. But I chose to stick around and take the brutal energy to protect Tippet. The treatment of that amazing dog created a major gap between us. It also altered my approach with his younger son because he also teased Tippet. I already disliked his brother due to some of the things he did, and what he said behind my back. But I was feeling sour towards him as well. He and his dad would call Tip names and tell him how ugly he was. I'd beg them to stop and it just egged them on. My partner would tell me that Tip's eyes were popping out of his sockets; that he was so ugly, he was cute. It was soul-crushing, because I knew by the look in Tippet's eyes that he understood. My partner would counter with, "He's just a dog." Then he'd follow by insisting that they didn't know words; they only knew tones. Again, that wasn't true.

They absolutely knew, "Good morning," as that was our activation call to create something wonderful. They understood, "Let's go outside – ride – walk – hike – and treat." They responded to, "No – good boy – and good girl" – and could distinguish between, "Let me see your tummy – stretchy – and I'll be back." Tippet especially knew that last one because it made him so sad. But once I'd return, he'd completely forget about it. They connected with, "I love you," the most because there weren't enough times in the day that I could say it to them. They were keen on their nicknames – "Charbar – Charbees – Princess – Tip – Tips – and Tippers" – and the energy behind them. They knew plenty of words, commands, and patterns, and my partner knew it. He just ran out of ways to justify being a dick to Tippet.

Over time, stories would come out of how my partner used to despise those dogs. He'd try to act like he didn't know what anybody was talking about. But it was blatant that he was not an animal lover. He didn't encompass that type of compassion for pets. He was more of an egotist who knew everything and had the biggest everything. In his mind, he was never wrong, it was never his fault, and he was the injured duck. When in reality, it was all a front. From who beat him up him as a kid – who wronged him as an adult – how his ex-wife used him – how his ex-girlfriend did the same – how people stole money from him – and how coaches ostracized him – I'd have to hear about "poor him." He especially painted a ruthless picture of his ex-wife, although her and I got along just fine. He admitted that he felt bad for the mean things he used to say to her. But then I'd hear that he cheated on her. It seemed like he fabricated sagas in order to keep me divided from her and everyone else who knew who he really was.

As year three came into the rotation, I started to hit rock-bottom. It was the beginning of the pandemic so, in a way, I wasn't alone. I had already been thrown out, and/or told to pack up, eight times. I also foolishly came back and/or unpacked eight times. By then, I absolutely hated living with him, being around any part of him, and having to see or hear him. I didn't have a word to say to him, his jokes were obnoxious, and I wanted to throw up every time he touched me. He was someone who intentionally destroyed parts of my human component. I didn't have anywhere to go and just prayed to be saved. The problem was that I was hinged to him. He wasn't ever going to let me out of his life with those dogs in my possession. So, I began the ninth cycle by continuing to put up with all the mayhem once again.

From the beginning of March until August, we spent our entire time in the mountains at a piece of property we had purchased in July of that previous year from his parents. Due to the financial backing of my mom, we were able to make that happen. Upon that sale, we had already launched a complete renovation on the place beginning with refurnishing and redecorating the cabin and garage. Just as Spring was about to roll in, we continued with remodeling and upgrading the entire twenty or so acres of pristine terrain. The place became stunning and, for the first time, I felt a hint of security.

I had been reluctant to acquire that place as a real estate investment a year earlier because of the negative energy that came with it. My partner had told me countless stories of the family turmoil that he had experienced there while growing up. It just seemed like bad karma. What sold me was the golf course lawn in the middle of the mountains and the almost two miles of sparkling waterfront along the frontside of the cabin. You could wake up early in the morning and catch a deer drinking from the river. It also helped that the land was home to a mom and daughter pair of majestic horses. That was an aspect of nature I had been missing while living in Los Angeles.

After all the hard work, and seeing how beautiful it turned out, I knew we made a great investment. Plus, the time, energy, and effort became therapeutic. For one, it separated me from him. I didn't have to walk with caution, have my phone snooped through, or listen to his same old music. The experience also gave me more alone time with the dogs, including an adorable furry friend owned by one of the neighbors up the road. His name was "Blue" and we had met him the previous summer when he was just a puppy. As with all animals, he came right up to me. He was the most radiant little playful guy with mesmerizing sky-blue white eyes. The dogs loved him and he loved them. It was like they say, "A match made in heaven!"

In the time we were out there, Blue had blossomed into a much bigger and robust leader. Yet, he was still extremely loving. His playful demeanor hadn't changed one bit. I could tell that he had adjusted to the role of his kingdom, because he knew those mountains better than anyone. Brilliant Blue had officially become a country dog!

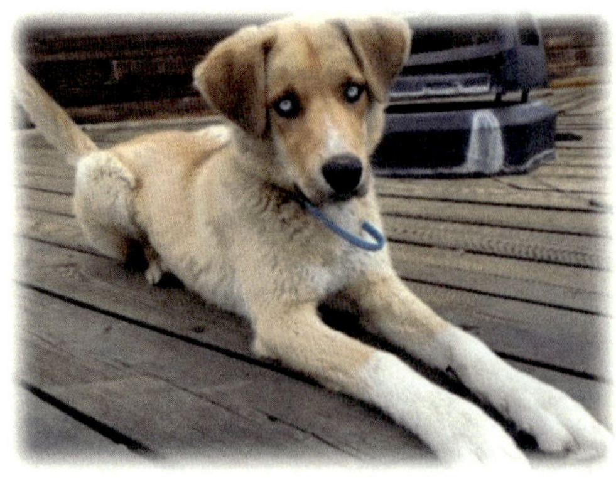

He would come eat with us, run to where we were at, hike with us, play in the rain, and would always sleep out on our front deck waiting for another chance to do it all over again. When I'd be in the tractor for over eight hours a day cutting the bushes, both of my dogs would either be sitting on my lap, or outside along my route running rampant with Blue. Every time we'd drive off the property, he would race by the truck so that he could safely see us off. I knew there was something magical about him. It was as if he was another one of my spirit animals and we were there to make the world a better place. Being anywhere around him, and seeing how enlightened him and my dogs were together, was euphoric. What a peaceful escape that was.

As with all other happy times, my partner persisted in shattering them between Blue and I. I'd get scolded for feeding him any food, much less scraps, as well as putting a rug out on the deck for him to sleep on. Since he couldn't get rid of him, he decided to start shooting innocent critters to supposedly keep them from ruining the land. He just told me that to justify him and his son killing animals for fun. His best friend was also staying on the property and joined in by shooting a Magpie one day. I couldn't bear the thought of what those poor creatures had to go through, so I distanced myself even more.

I remember the moment I found the bird. I was taking a walk down to the river with Char and Tip and noticed him laying on the ground with a hole through his heart. From then on, everything shifted. Energies became even more aggressive and sarcastic towards me, and Tip ended up getting attacked by his buddy Blue. It was like a curse had been placed on us, or at least on me.

I had given all three dogs a bone, like always, and separated them. Within seconds, I heard a fierce commotion. Then, Tippet was at the front door covered in grass. He looked like he was in shock. It turned out that Blue had taken a bite out of his neck and parts of his limbs. As I laid there with him, I tried to comfort his scared little self. I saw that he had a hole in his neck like the Magpie did in his heart. Later that evening, I picked him up in his doggy bed and took him to the guest room so that Char and I could sleep close to him. By the next morning, he was back outside playing with Blue. Those are dogs for you; one moment they're in a mind zone, and the next, they forget.

My partner used that incident as a tool to separate me from Blue and instantly halted our interactions. From that day on, he was never allowed back. My partner treated him like a convicted killer for hurting Tippet the way he did. I knew that it was all just an act and another one of his malicious maneuvers. He chased Blue off the land by screaming at him, shot his gun in the area of his ears without a care if he went deaf, and advised the neighbor to keep him off the property. I could tell that Blue was entirely perplexed. That was the only way of life he knew. The neighbor was so intimidated of my partner, that on the next occasion Blue trespassed onto the acreage, he grabbed him by the neck, held him down, and appeared to break his leg. That scream has haunted me to this day.

I missed Blue more than ever and I could tell that the dogs did too. We'd continue to roam the land and see him up on top of the hill looking down at us in complete sadness. It was heartbreaking to hear him howl in the middle of the night as if crying in pain. With the loss of Blue, I could feel another piece of my soul getting clawed out. I was cracking like the crust of Crème Brulee and wilting away like the pedals of a dead flower. All I could do was continue to give Charly and Tippet everything I had left. As difficult as it was to go on without Blue, we had to. We did it in his honor, for the time we were blessed to share with him, and for the love we would always have for him.

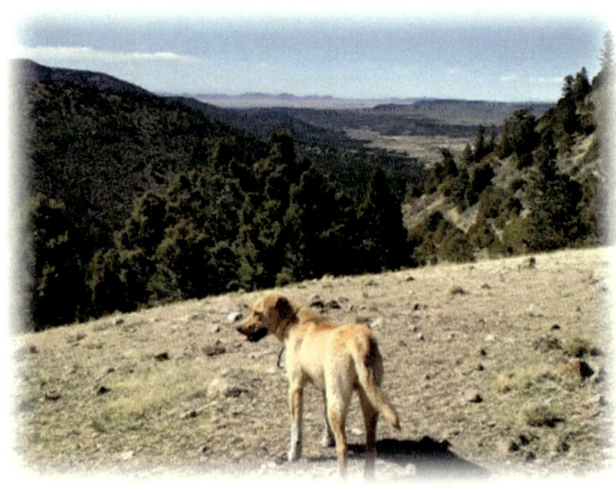

The dogs and I would go down to the river and dam together, watch the water sparkle and the fish swim by together, meditate together, pull positive guidance cards together, engage in nature together, play in the dirt together, and graze in the sun together. When my partner was out doing his own thing, we'd relax on the cushioned patio couch and watch the beautiful hummingbirds devour the sugar water from our feeders. When we would drive up to the higher lakes to fish, they would follow my path and, even at times, get in the water to be closer. When we'd go hiking, they'd explore places they never could imagine. It was so meaningful to watch them inspect and analyze every single tree, rock, grass, and elk shed.

When we were back at the cabin, they would sit on the floor with me and place their paws on some part of my legs. They just had to touch me to feel safe, especially Charly. She always needed to be right next to me. My partner detested it so much that he would pick her up and take her away because he wanted her to lay close to him on the couch. She would immediately growl and, within a few minutes, be right back on the floor touching some part of my leg. He could never grasp the fact that he couldn't force them to love him the way they loved me. He surely couldn't buy them like he bought everyone else.

Since he knew he couldn't get the upper edge by stealing Charly, he went back to picking on Tippet. Both up in the mountains and back at home, he pestered and heckled him. That became his way of continually puncturing me. A month after the attack, we had to be in the metro area for a few days to take care of some business inquiries. We decided to take the dogs for a usual walk through the neighborhood. As we rounded the last corner, we noticed that one of the entitled neighbors had left her two horrible Shih Tzus off their leashes. They immediately charged at Charly and Tippet. I was holding Char on the leash and my partner was holding Tip on his. I immediately nudged her away because they were going to go at it. My partner, on the other hand, allowed one of those mini monsters to lunge and attack Tippet. Before we knew it, Tip was on his back, tangled in his leash, and screaming for help. The dog had pinned him to the side of the curb with his mouth in Tip's neck.

It was as if my partner intentionally allowed that to happen. Tippet had become powerless. As quickly as I could, I kicked that little monster just enough to get him off of Tip. Then I instantly picked him up. The owner stayed calm while sitting on her front porch laughing. Talk about another reminder of the repulsive frequency around me. Instead of comforting Tip's mind and heart, from then on, my partner felt the need to laugh at the incident and call him a "pussy." It became another blow I tried to digest. Seeing the mental trauma that it was causing poor little Tippers was harrowing.

Aside from the pandemonium, we were back in the mountains a few days later and the dogs and I would continue to be inseparable. We were kindred spirits and nobody could deny that. Even my partner's own friends and family witnessed our strong bond in the city as well as when they came to visit us at the cabin. I truly believed that those dogs were the reason I returned back to my hometown. We were brought together so that I could make up for all I didn't do with my previous pets when I was a kid. In turn, it would allow me to give them everything with ample love as an adult. They knew it. They were well aware that wherever I would go, they would go with me. Although we had been separated for eight cycles of death, there would never be a time again when we would be apart. I reassured them every minute of every day that there was nothing to worry about. We would lay together on the floor and look into each other's eyes. And every time, I would make that promise to them.

On a bright Sunday daybreak that second week of August, all three of us went outside to attempt to work out. I was saggy, hideous looking, aged, tired, weathered, and just felt like junk. I figured that I might as well try to revive my cells and attempt to get back into a decent enough shape to feel good. I had already been robbed of the belief I had in myself, my dreams, career aspirations, personal objectives, and any hope for a happy future. Add over twenty pounds of dead weight and you'd get an idea of how much more unappealing I felt. Something just told me to go outside and try to sweat out the overwhelmingly heavy energy. I could tell the dogs were up for it as well. We gathered our weights, iPod, jump rope, yoga mat, and water, and headed out to enjoy the beautiful open-air biosphere.

As we were leaving, I took one last glance inside. My partner looked upset like always. I figured it was another one of his moody days like every damn day. He hadn't said a word to me up to that point, but I still asked him if he wanted to exercise with me. Of course, he said, "No." Within a few minutes, he and his son decided to drive into town. It was a blessing to get a few hours of tranquility with the dogs, and not have to spend my morning hearing one of his usual insults that I "talked too much."

By the time they returned, we were hanging out down by the river. I didn't know if it was a coincidence or synchronicity, but Blue came running up to us at that exact moment. I had longed so much to hug him, and now I had the chance to. Tippet and Charly were excited to see him as well. He rolled around and snuggled up to Tip while Charly barked at him like she always did at every onset. It was hilarious and just like old times. There was no love lost between those dogs. I didn't even think twice about the consequences. I just enjoyed being present with all three of them.

Surprisingly, my partner decided to join us. He was walking our way with his fishing pole, and looked to be fine with Blue there. As he got closer, there was fury on his face. He didn't say a word, marched right by, and casted his line into the water. I took a few steps towards him and softly explained that Blue just wanted to play for a minute, and that I'd make sure to steer him off shortly. He yelled back, "I told you I didn't want that dog on the property!"

He threw his pole down and trudged off. I guided Blue away gently, and could actually see that he understood. He headed into the sunset in a way that I knew he'd be okay. It was like he came to say goodbye to me with hugs and kisses. It was such a reassuring moment.

The dogs and I walked up to the cabin and weren't inside for ten minutes before my partner came barging in. Foam was bubbling out of the corner creases of his mouth. He got in my face and told me to "pack my shit and get the fuck out of his house." Time may not stop for anyone. But in that instant, it did for me. He began ripping frames off the walls, décor from the shelves, and throwing them on the floor. Then he went into the garage to get some plastic storage boxes, and flung them into the bedroom while having a few choice words for me.

Charly and Tippet were frozen with fear. I could see the sadness taking over their pupils. They knew what was happening. I walked into the bathroom and began packing. It was my 9th eviction and I didn't have much left. Just as I was done boxing up my things, I looked up and asked if the dogs could come while I moved out of the home we shared in the city? Surprisingly, he nodded, "Yes."

We began driving off the property, when Blue magically appeared and ran alongside as he always did. He had a bit of a limp, but nothing was going to stop him from seeing me off with the most abundant love. I locked eyes with his beautiful cobalts, saw his illuminating smile, and felt his essence. I rolled down the window, and as I waved goodbye to another soulmate, I smiled and mouthed the words, "I love you," to him. That was the last time I'd ever see my Blue again.

We made the three-hour trip back home in complete silence. Charly laid in my arms the entire time and Tippet burrowed in between the side of my thigh and the console. When we pulled up to the house, my partner launched the garage door open and threw my bags and boxes on the floor. Then he drove off. I had no idea the journey I'd have ahead of me. In that moment, all I could feel was a pleasant haze of love knowing that I'd get a few more days with the dogs. I had nowhere to go, no money, and no resources to move. Yet, I had them... and that was all that mattered.

For the next four days, I spent every moment I could with them. As I packed clothes, crystals, and what was left of the Zen room, I'd reach over and cuddle their little faces, give them kisses, and tell them how much I loved them. My partner had actually notified me that I could bring them to my mom's house that weekend for my parents to say goodbye. I still didn't think he'd really take them away from me. He knew that separating us would be detrimental to them, especially to Charly. He also knew that I would die for them. But that was his ammo So, it wasn't a surprise when he texted me in those last hours demanding that I leave them. My gut kept telling me to go for it. Then, like so many previous times, I went against it. I didn't know if he'd harm them if he ever found us. He had knocked down doors, kicked a dog off a bed, pulled out a gun, and ripped Char and Tip out of my arms several times. There was no telling what he would do.

They always loved a plain hamburger patty from McDonald's. So, on our last day, we headed out for one final treat. I'll never forget looking at the anticipation in their eyes not having any idea that I'd be leaving them. As we got back to the house, I felt like my feet were welding into the hot cement. Each step got heavier and slower. We walked in and they were excitedly jumping around. What an awful feeling I had in my stomach knowing that I was going to have to trick them. I placed the meat on their plates and they immediately began devouring it. In that instant, I held whatever breath I had left, and raced out the back. I remember Charly looking up at me with a glimpse of panic. I slammed the door, hit the garage button, and watched it close that life-enhancing connection. I had never gasped for air as much as I did in those seconds.

How was I going to live with myself by misleading them so that they'd be distracted? How was I going to go on after breaking my promise that we'd never be apart? I knew I probably wouldn't ever get those answers, but it was the only way I could do it. I wasn't able to sit down with them and say goodbye. I wasn't able to look into their eyes and tell them how much I loved them, how much better they made me, and how much I already missed them. I wasn't able to hold them in my arms one last time for one last kiss.

I never saw them again.

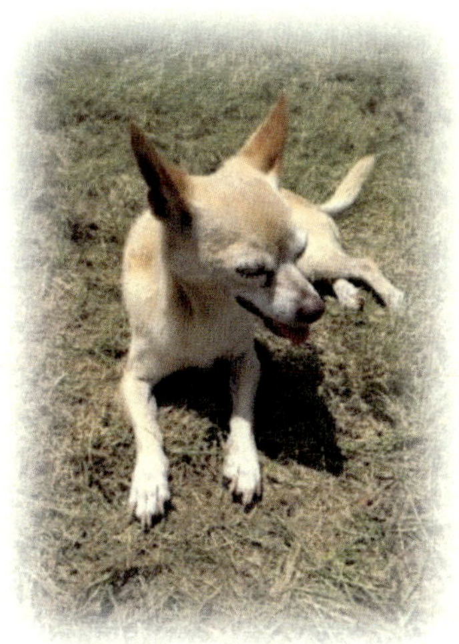

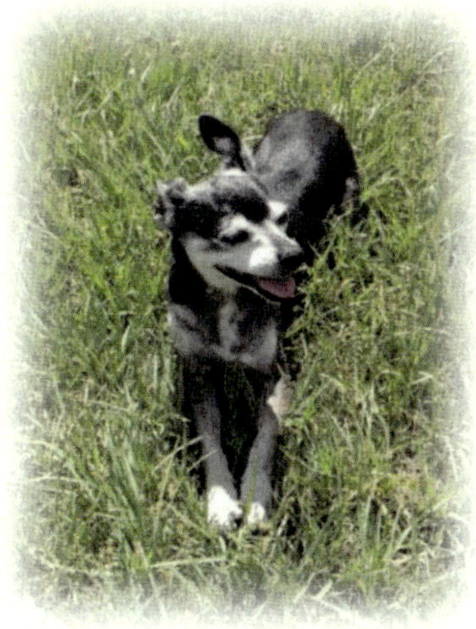

PART 2

Rebirth and the Three Moons

5
The Winds of Change

They say that the number "9" represents completion. In two years, I had been told to leave eight times and a final 9th the third year… on the 9th day of that August. I had nowhere to go, very little belongings, hardly any residuals coming in, no job or dogs, and in the middle of a global pandemic. I had lost all aspects of what I encompassed, hope for any happiness, and the effervescence for life in general. If I thought I was in trouble after the first five months of my romance, then I was really screwed. Maybe that "9" meant the end of my life and I was coming back home to die. Trust that it sure did feel like it.

I had returned to a place I never really appreciated while growing up, as I had been relocated to the mountains on my mom and stepdad's 3-acre property. I knew they had adored every aspect of residing out there for most of their relationship, but I just couldn't align with it. Toilets didn't get flushed, the water came from a community well, and you had to place your tissue wipings in the trash can instead of flushing them. Yards were bombarded with junk and broken-down vehicles; some with wiring that had been infested by rats and mice. Others, were missing parts and rotted out from the weather. Stray dogs were either homeless and starving, or homed, roaming around barking all night. They were so vicious that you couldn't take a walk, or jog, anywhere in the vicinity. If that wasn't scary enough, you could hear the coyotes howling in a high-pitched intensity when the nighttime blanketed the sky. Weeds grew everywhere and Chamizo bushes, foxtails, cacti, and Juniper trees lined the properties. Flies, ants, and mosquitos annoyingly rotated with the seasons… and dust, wind, allergies, dry air, and continuous years of droughts were the norm. That wind definitely made an ongoing statement because, every time I complained about it, things just seemed to keep me even more planted.

Nonetheless, being forty minutes from town and an hour and a half from the metro city meant having to travel on a highway lathered with roadkill and Descansos. Those were shrines of crosses and flowers in memoriam from fatal wreckages. It was literally like driving through an ongoing graveyard. With every trip back and forth, it seemed like they would multiply. Maybe that was because those structured tributes brought back a constant reminder of the nonfunctioning energy of my past relationship. I swear, everywhere we would go together – whether it be somewhere around the city for a softball game, work, or leisure, or driving up for a scenic getaway in the mountains – I'd see cemeteries. I knew I was being sent messages when I was with him that something was killing my spirit.

My parents were simple creatures by nature. They never needed anything excessive, and especially didn't take the outdoors for granted. Although they lived in two separate homes on the property as companions, they maintained their connectedness with an absolute love for that area and all it represented. I'd like to think that I had a similar mentality in not needing material things to define me. As a child, we were a middle-income household with my mom going to school and working three jobs to support us. Due to my dad's disabling heart issues, he was steered into being a stay-at-home parent. He made sure to make everything so exciting that I never thought we were any less than rich.

I still dabbled in dreams of big city lights, money, fancy clothes, and travel that many youngsters did at that age. But I'm sure that had a lot to do with my father instilling various levels of ambition in me. I also learned early on to make the best out of anything. Then I headed to college and began my initial experience with traveling. I was introduced to a whole new lifestyle that, by the time I shipped off to LA, I had already manifested the illusions of what I felt identified me. After a few internal deaths and a few internal rebirths, I returned to that little kid who didn't need all that superficial fluffy stuff. I had entered the middle stage of adulthood as my mature authentic self. I just thought that due to the hardship I was going through, and losing so much of who I was, that I was unable to see anything remotely positive.

Fortunately, one of the projects my ex and I had accomplished during the first year of our relationship was the renovation and remodel of my mom's mobile home. She had taken the trailer over from her previous tenants who put zero effort into caring for it and, in fact, thrashed it. Initially, I thought we got in way over our heads. After a complete gutting of the inside and the addition of new paint, wood flooring, design, and décor, the place turned into a showroom that could've landed in an interior design magazine. It was absolutely stunning. I may have been in a dark hole during that period, but that venture had been something I was very proud of. I managed to fit what I had left in the newly built added extra bedroom, which measured to be approximately 10x10 feet. For my entire stay, that room would be my thrown.

In the first month of my new temporary residence, I was in complete shock. I had just tricked Charly and Tippet in a way so that I could make a clean getaway. That guilt was eating me alive along with the grueling sadness and pain I harbored from losing them. I spent most of the time just trying to clot the open bleeding wounds. I cried daily without having any control over the timing of the outbursts, and just couldn't understand how or why I'd be put through so much agony. I didn't care about my ex, and didn't have a single concern of whether or not he was equally affected. I had already become aware of his fake character and had grown extremely angry. What I thought I knew, though, would turn out to only be a minuscule of his manipulation. When more truths would eventually come to the forefront, I would become inundated in the "whys" of my entire life.

Before it could really sink in, his father passed away. I proclaimed my absence from that service, as I was just beginning to feel a bit better. Yet, how could I not show up? His father and I had shared such a meaningful connection that it would be a disservice to him and all he constituted. After speaking with my mom, I decided to put everything aside for that small window, and do the right thing in respect and honor of such a wonderful man that I loved so dearly.

We parked and walked towards the setup only to see my ex standing there as if psychically waiting for us. It was like I just couldn't shed the bad luck. I had already dumped a few pounds from crying them off, but that was ridiculous. I was an internal wreck to say the least. Yet, in that moment, I gathered myself as best as I could and buckled up.

He approached the three of us like a good old boy that he wasn't and acted like nothing had happened. As outraged as my parents were with him, they held their composure and offered their condolences. Then they strolled off to give us a minute. Once they were far enough away not to hear his garbage, he began verbally attacking me about why I didn't call him. Then he threw in something about "having to do what he did to me in order to set me free."

All I could think of was how did I expect to show up to that funeral without him badgering me? He continued rambling on so much that I didn't even remember anything else after that, until he stopped and stared at me with hollow eyes. I waited for his next reason for why I supposedly did him wrong. Instead, with a deadpan glare and a flattened tone, he said, "You know, Blue got dragged for two miles."

I practically lost the stability of my legs and all control of my tears, and my heart sank to the bottom of the pavement.

He said, "A truck forgot that he'd been tied to the back of it and dragged him up part of the canyon."

With all the strength I had, I said to him, "Why would you tell me that?"

He replied, "I thought you'd want to know."

I put my sunglasses on as tears poured down my face, swallowed the last of my saliva, and began to crawl away. How I made it more than a few strides was beyond me. Then, like always, he said he was sorry. I had been separated from him for over a month and by almost a hundred miles, and he was still trying to hurt me by ripping my guts out in a matter of a few sentences. I actually remained cordial with him throughout the rest of the service. But what a mistake I made for showing up that morning. I had worked so hard in that month to try and get to a place where I could see five feet in front of me. And now, it was all reoccurring. Sadly, I'd come to find out that it was only the beginning. Not only did he remove life from me, but it would surface that he also deceived me out of the investments we made when we were together; also deceiving my mother.

During our courtship, we had put money into a few private companies and purchased real property in hopes of securing a financial future together. Two of those major opportunities became possible through the financial backing of my mother. One included the mountain property I had previously spent many months helping to renovate and upgrade in value. Much of the work had been completed with a high-end tractor and truck that were purchased in my name and under my credit. The remodeling amenities were purchased by a credit card also taken out in my name and credit. This was the same property I was thrown out of. Another happened to be a startup of one we had already put money into the previous year.

We couldn't have purchased the country acreage or invested the amount we did without my mom's help. Come to find out, he used the funds for himself; placing everything solely in his name and new LLC that I wasn't listed on. The deal was that he'd pay back one loan in installation payments, and get the other paid off through a real-estate contract. It was never agreed that I'd be excluded. My mom and I had trusted that he was doing the right thing. Talk about getting used and taken advantage of for our lack of knowledge.

The Universe worked in strange ways because, soon after those unveilings, he left me a voice message. I had no interest in calling back, but it was apparent that he needed help in a legal case that he got my mom involved in. Not only was his company getting sued for alleged negligent work, but so was her agency for referring him to the same high-end client. He began asking me what kind of information I provided as if I was going to put up my paws and save him. Instead, I began screaming at him for throwing me out with nothing, and betraying me. He calmly replied that he was sorry and shouldn't have handled things the way he did. But he'd done a lot for my parents, so he didn't owe me any money. He accused me of abusing him and told me that I was depressed. I don't know how it got to us spending the day speaking on the phone amicably. But then I realized that it was a ploy to reel me back in. I let him know that I was done and to please leave me be. He agreed, but made sure to finish the conversation by thanking me for teaching him how to love a dog, as Charly was now "his little girl." I hung up and spent the night in a flood of tears.

That call and those findings would bring about a new layer of regret and resentment, not to mention nightmares. I'd have horrible dreams of my ex purposely sabotaging me. They would involve him publicly humiliating me, destroying any chances at success, and taking Charly and Tippet away from me. Even more disturbing, would be both dogs gruesomely dying, fading away, or being forgotten about. In one dream, parts of Tippet's body were falling on the ground, in pieces, right in front of me, and I was desperately trying to put him back together. I just wanted to save him. I hated those visuals and the panic I'd wake up with. They made it tough to find any peace in my day, especially thinking that they were dying without me. I was already submerged in a back-and-forth motion of shock, anger, sadness, guilt, and fear. Add to that, feeling lost, empty, and confused.

I began thinking that it had to do with how I felt about myself and the attachment to the decision I made three years earlier to change my life. Maybe it wasn't about what he did to me, but more about going against my gut. Maybe my dreams were telling me that it was me I desperately wanted to put back together, and the one who needed to be saved. I kept asking myself why I stayed in such a volatile situation. Why didn't I just leave??? I remembered telling a few of my clients those same famous words. I'd emphasize how unhealthy the toxicity was, not to forget who they were, and that they deserved better. I finally understood that it wasn't that easy.

I never thought I'd be in the same position. It sounds cliché, but you don't see it coming. By the time you do, it's too late. They're pros at the conning game. They begin by concealing their identities and pretending to be what you think you're attracted to. Then they show their supposed vulnerable sides and, now, you want to help them. All the while, they're manipulating you by doing nice things and being on their best behavior. But they're just edging closer to owning you.

That's partly how they lure you in the first place, and my ex did do a lot of nice things. He gave me a break from LA, provided me with a rent-free home, gym membership, organic food, covered my bills, paid for expensive allergy treatments, bought me cool stuff, and took care of the remaining grand on my school loan. Since my car was the only vehicle that we used for almost a year into our relationship, he also paid off what I owed. He taught me how to build things, construct homes, and renovate landscapes. We traveled, gambled, fished, played tennis, golfed, hiked, and remodeled. We also helped each other's parents and enjoyed some really funny times.

The benefits came with a catch, though. And it meant being infested with supervision, isolation, jealousy, verbal bashing, extreme mood swings, and a constant portrayal of the "poor me syndrome." He'd forcibly insist on paying for everything. Then he'd accuse everyone of using him for money, and not being compensated for work he offered as a gift, or in exchange for services. The daily constriction made me feel like I was stuck in quicksand; slowly suffocating me from my bottom half up. I couldn't do anything about it because I was drained of everything. In turn, I became dependent on him for everything. I hated myself, all I ever loved, and didn't have an ounce of a bright outlook. The paralysis moved up my body due to no longer having goals or visions and, for sure, no motivation. Since money was his primary means of control, I had to leave the ring, and wasn't given a dime, every time he kicked me out. I had nowhere to go, so I sucked it up and continued taking the mental torment.

I know there were some good things about him, and deep down inside, he had some kind qualities. He just lacked self-love and it became apparent that his way of fulfillment was to bring others down with him. The bad easily outweighed the good and it eventually became detrimental to my psyche. Thank goodness he threw me out as deplorable as he did. Otherwise, I don't know if I would've ever left. I can say today, that I will never again judge anyone for experiencing any form of an emotionally destructive encounter, whether short term or long term, and not walking away. That is a promise I can keep.

After the mind cluster began to fizzle into another form of self-interrogation, all I could come up with as to the purpose and positives were Charly and Tippet. I felt that we were brought together into that pestilent vortex so that I could elevate their spiritual connection and life adventures. I also felt it was the link I needed in giving me another chance. Whether it was designed to renew their lives and extend their quality of experience, or for them to revive mine and extend me the same blessings, the three of us were meant to be.

We had such a powerful pact that on the days my ex would throw me out of the house, I could see a little piece of death in both of their eyes. Charly, at one point, even suddenly got sick. We couldn't figure out why, and it seemed like the doctors were just as baffled. After bouts with several different medications and a blessed second opinion, we were able to align her with the exact 3-day treatment that helped get her pancreas functioning back to normal. It wouldn't be until after my final separation that I'd realize she also stored her emotional trauma in that same part of her digestive tract as I did.

That day, she and I laid out on the front lawn together after picking her up from the emergency room. Her head strength was slightly returning, but I felt it was just enough for me to receive her message. I could see that she was giving up her life so that I could leave and regain my own. I knew that she would stick around long enough to make sure Tippet was okay. But I felt she was ready to go so that I could go back home. She was so strong that she would die for me. In the end, I stayed for both of them. In the end, I lost them.

I had placed a few pictures of some of my best memories with them on my vision boards. I truly believed that I could manifest them back into my arms for good. Yet, it wasn't happening. My mom had made attempts to contact my ex asking to please give them back, but he never budged. By that time, my hope began to fade. I knew I would never be the same without them. A part of me would be hallow, and a part of me would be better because of them.

My parents also missed Charly and Tippet with all of their hearts. There was such a sweet friendship between them. I know they were just as pained, but they had other pets to help take their minds off the sadness. My mom, and especially my stepdad, were always fond of animals and rescued plenty throughout the decades. They had a rotation of dogs, cats, goats, a friendly wild pigeon, nearby rabbits, hummingbirds, and saved several feathered creatures. That wasn't common because, in those rural areas, people had a whole different take on animals. Rather than saving them, there was a large hunting community who was more about the sport and mounting heads and horns on their living room walls. They'd also eat cow tongues and throw barbeques in celebration of slaughtering innocent pigs.

There were locals who were rumored to run cock fights and others who bred and prepped dogs for fighting rings, not to mention selling puppies for thousands. Some would even steal people's pets and use them as bait dogs. There were households known to neglect their chickens, rabbits, and sheep to the point that they'd get ripped apart from the same neighboring mutts. Pets were left changed outside, 24/7, in the freezing cold and sweltering heat. There were plenty of folks who shouldn't have been allowed to own or be around any animals as you'd find them shot and dumped for no reason at all.

Not only were lost, abandoned, scared, starving darlings everywhere, but you'd also see dried up emaciated cattle and horses on nearby reservations trying to find water. They'd be embedded under the one tree that could've helped save them from the desert climate. It reminded me of the dire culture of the mountain community I had just experienced in my partnership. One such atrocity was big money clientele paying top dollar to sit in their vehicles while trappers had their hounds chase bears and mountain lions up trees... only to shoot dead the defenseless animals for game. The lack of ethical treatment and disregard for sentient beings was heart-wrenching. It was no different and just as disturbing where I was currently living.

When I arrived that second week of August, my parents currently had three rescue dogs and a feral cat all aged in the double digits. They also had a female puppy that they came across a year earlier after finding her in the middle of the frontage rood bloody and injured. She was a special something for my parents as well as for Charly and Tippet. They had met her when she was much smaller, and their interactions were always adorable. She had grown into a much fuller dog by that point, but would turn out to be the sweetest, loving little girl. She was especially good with Charly and Tippet when they'd come to visit and the times when my parents dog sat for us.

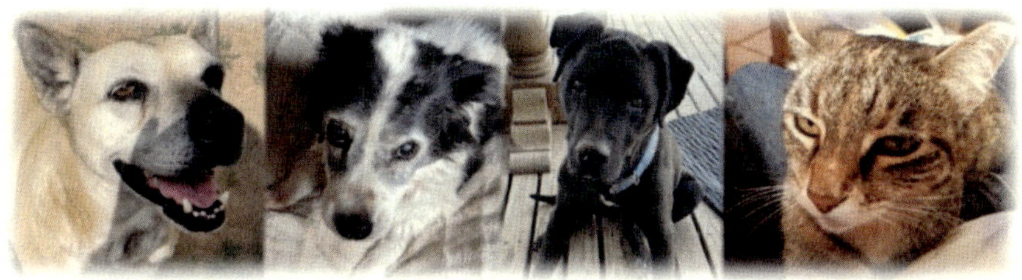

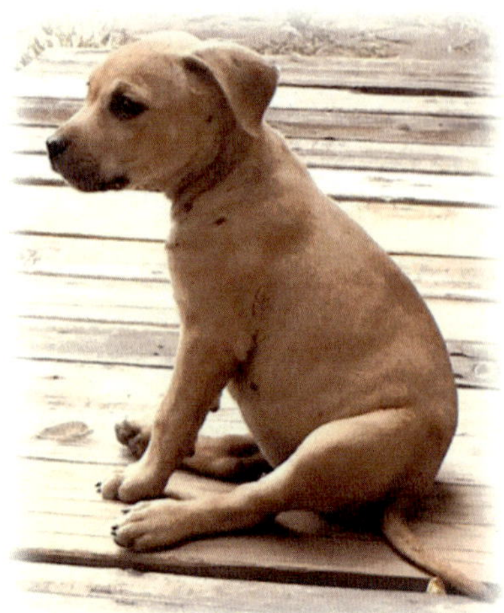

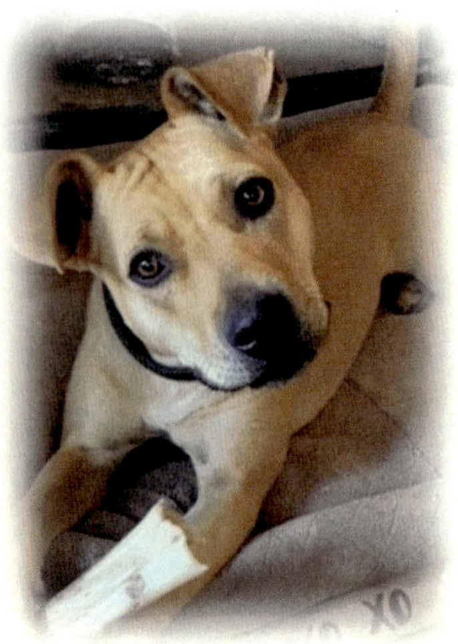

"Goldie" would be a tremendous pillar in the next coming months, as being around her all day would spark a bit of strength back into my own legs. I actually began to make some decent progress. That's how I knew I wasn't completely at the point of destitution. I was able to do my best to take care of all the work around the property, the manual labor my parents weren't physically capable of doing, any building and construction, all technical issues with phones, televisions, and computers, managing their accounts, and my own take on creativity and design in rejuvenating their outdoor grounds.

My mom would work all day and I'd make sure the house was always clean and maintained. I'd help my stepdad with whatever he needed in his area. And by the time my mom arrived home, the three of us would watch sporting games and enjoy having dinner together. The quality of those moments with them was something I hadn't experienced since I transferred colleges to finish my last two years closer to home. We would rotate every Sunday between myself, my dad, my mom and stepdad, and my stepbrother, as the host for our family, sports, feast, and gambling day. I had jetted off to New York. And then right after I got my degree, I headed to LA where my only visits would become 2-week vacations during the holidays.

It was nice to see the formula those two had developed after all the years. They would finish each other's sentences, believed the same media propaganda, supported the same politicians, loved music and sports, and enjoyed drinking a couple of beers after a day of pulling weeds. My mom had been gradually losing her hearing for the past five or six years, but they still managed to understand every component of each other's systems. It was amazing to watch them navigate so well together. I was getting to know them on a whole different level; not just as my parents, but as my friends. I could see how happy me being there made them. The only things missing were Charly, Tippet, and my dad.

There were good days, or I should say, "better days." And there were days that were worse than all others before. On those better days, I would put more affirmations on my vision boards, and then go outside and sit in silence as the breeze blew comfort onto my face. It was a surreal simple place of solace for me. In the midst of the most debilitating storm of my life, I was finding some sense of calmness. I hated who I was, how I got where I got, that I had nothing left, and how my dogs were taken away from me. Yet, I was somewhat calm.

Where was I in a such rush to get to anyway, and how could I get there? The entire world was locked down. I couldn't travel, get a job, or do much of anything except get to know myself and my soul again. I was 46 years of age living back home with my parents, and all I could do was try my best to have a good day and be at peace with the present moment. I may not have understood it or been able to accept any of it. But thankfully, I was able to see some sort of positive light; primarily in the joy I brought to my 71-year-young parents. Although I cried through much of it, I journaled every day, meditated, EFT tapped, and posted inspirational messages on social media. The wind was shifting the direction for me. And for once, I wasn't in a hurry.

6
The Bodhi Tree

It was a freezing cold December morning in single digit degrees and snowcapped trees. Winter was upon us and actually very beautiful to see nature covered in a sheer white comforter. I laid there in bed, cozied up in three layers of blankets thinking about how I was going to try and revive my life. I had to move, not so much in residence. But yes, that too. I had to start becoming mobile again in body and in mind. I hadn't written as much as I should've, sharpened my memory and acting skills, practiced my vocal exercises, or used my brain for anything. I had become the new handyman out at my parent's property, so I was earning my rent-free living through manual labor. LOL! Yet, it took all I had to motivate myself enough to ride the stationary bike, much less run a mile and lift a weight.

I knew that the only way I could get my motor running was to do something that scared me. Never had I believed that it took fear or discomfort to be successful. Those societal programs were conditioned into our minds the same way as "no pain, no gain" manifested in gyms. In my previous experiences, overexertion did more harm than good, and hadn't been my means of advancement on any level. I was in one of the blurriest periods of my life and realized that in order to regain my focus, I was going to have to do something that forced me out of my comfort zone. Otherwise, I was going to become complacent and end up settling again.

My parents had furnished me with an abundance of love, support, financial security, food, laughter, and the "me time" that I so badly needed. They were salts of the earth who would've provided me that safe, loving setting forever, and did all they could to sway me to stay just as long. But I missed my solemn environment. It was vital to return to a place of my own where I could put myself back together, or at least try. I just wanted to make sure not to be in a rush and make impulsive decisions, especially since my Third Eye was so foggy.

Then one day, I got on Facebook. Many of the pages I liked and followed were animal and adoption affiliated. So, it wasn't a surprise that the first post was a picture of the most adorable little guy up for grabs. A dog was the last thing I had in mind. But for some reason, he captured my attention more than any others before him. His name was "Cody" and he was a scrawny little slightly bull-legged cream thing with folded ears, a pink collar, and the type of sadness in his eyes that could make an entire continent cry. I had seen tons of shelter dogs up for adoption in the four months I had been living with my parents and never did I think I'd rescue one. My main mission was sharing their mugshots with all of my friends and fans so that I could connect them with the homes and families that could.

The more I looked at his picture, the more I felt something so loving, adoring, and cosmic. I had to ask myself if this was the move I needed to make? Was this the fear I needed to face? I didn't own much, didn't have a solid source of income, and didn't have a clear vision of where I'd end up in five months. Plus, the country was still on lockdown. I couldn't be so self-consumed with the healing of my own soul that it could potentially harm the healing of another's, especially a pet who was a 100% dependent. I had to truly consider if I was ready to bring a doggy into my heart and home (my mom's home) with no guarantees, or security, of how I'd take care of him.

My gut was bubbling and the circulation in my veins heated up like scorching lava. But it was more of an optimistic vibe rather than the previous wavelengths of denial. I knew he was the one. I just didn't know if I could make it happen. I looked over to my vision boards and saw my beloved Charly and Tippet staring at me with those light-filled lenses and glowing smiles. My heart sank as I thought to myself, "I could never replace them." They were my children and they were my everything. Life had been so deficient without them, and the only thing that kept me functioning were the memories we shared together. The guilt of letting them go and moving on made me nauseous for a few minutes. Then something shifted inside, and I told myself that it was okay to love again. I had to allow myself the freedom from something I couldn't control and turn it into something wonderful. Just like them, this little guy came to me for a reason.

Deep down, I had known I was never getting them back. But in that moment, I finally accepted it. I had probably been causing more mental calamity having to see their beautiful faces every day on those boards knowing that truth. I had counted the weeks since being without them and that day was seventy-two hours into the nineteenth. I just prayed that they had forgotten about me so that they weren't suffering the same slow death being without me... that I was from being without them. I knew they would die one day without being by their side, and that was tough to digest. Yet, despite how broken I felt, it was finally time to trudge forward. I had to pull myself out of the swamp and dry off, empty and alone.

Thank goodness I was doing much better than four months prior. But I still had to find the opening to my air valve so that I could revive my happiness. If it was meant to be, I had to trust that we would find our way back to each other. It's always easier said than done. But at that point, all I had left was faith. I laid there for a while with my lids closed, and tried to loosen the tightness in my pancreas by placing my hands on my Solar Plexus. I don't even remember feeling my heart beat. My life was about to change once again; I just didn't know in what direction. Nobody could've ever written a better script than what came from making that phone call five minutes later.

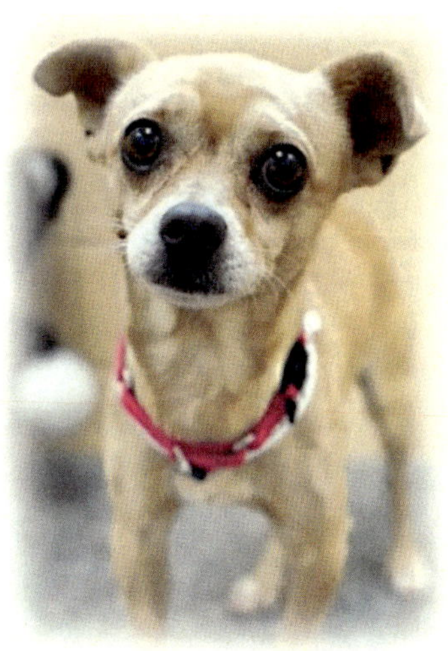

Funny enough, the dude wasn't even available. He had a long waiting list for potential new forever homes. Of course, he did. He was that magnetic! He was the cutest little creature in the world. Who wouldn't want to add him to their family? I asked if I could be put on the list anyway. I had to say, that in a sense, I was kind of glad it didn't work out. Panic had set in and I started overthinking that maybe it was too soon, and that I was jumping the gun. I hadn't even discussed it with my mom and didn't want to assume that she'd be okay with bringing another dog into her home. A pit rented space in my stomach. And for the rest of the weekend, I went with the flow and made the best of things.

That following Monday morning, I was driving on the frontage road on my way into town when, all of a sudden, a small Finch flew into my windshield. It was said that the surrounding wildfires had shifted the migration of birds. Not only were hundreds of thousands of them dying from the smoke, but many seemed to have lost their sense of perception. You'd constantly see them on the side of the road from crashing into cars. But why mine, and why on that day? It happened in such slow motion that I actually saw it coming as if pressing the pause button play-by-play on the television.

I immediately pulled over, picked up his lifeless body, and laid him down on a tree branch hidden from attackers. I told him how sorry I was and wished him blessings on his new journey, transformation, and destination. I had many encounters with animal and insect spirit totems throughout my life, especially at times when I needed their messages the most. Since being back in my hometown, roadrunners were the totems frequently showing up for me. I just had never killed one. I knew right then that something was coming to an end.

I carried on into town and ran the errands I set out to get done when the shelter called to say that Cody had become available again. They wanted to know if I was still interested. In that moment, the fear bubble didn't have a chance to shoot me down. I had to make a decision in a matter of seconds. So, I said, "Yes." She explained that I could come in for a meet-and-greet that Wednesday afternoon. We hung up and, for a few minutes, I stayed parked frozen with excitement!

Later that evening, I sat down with my parents to talk about Cody. I was prepared for them to say, "No." But surprisingly, they felt it would be a great move for me to make. They were pampering me and doing all they could in giving me the time it took for me to regain my happiness. They also didn't want me to fall into a spell of stagnation. Major responsibilities were on my horizon, as I would potentially have another mouth to feed. There was no way I was going to let my past experiences in a relationship hold me back and defeat me. I always had a gift for saving people, uplifting attitudes, and instilling self-confidence. Why couldn't I shift it to animals, and why couldn't we both win? Knowing that I was about to extend the quality of life for a dog felt like landing the perfect leading role alongside Andy Garcia. It was already that fulfilling!

That morning, without any guarantee that we'd be a good match, I decided to take down my pictures of Charly and Tippet... and write them a farewell letter. It was one of the most difficult things I ever had to do. I opened up my laptop and began entering that day in my journal. It felt like I was about to write an obituary; my last loving words to my children dying of cancer as I watched them slowly fade away in their hospital beds. Those two had such a strong bond together. And as crushing as it was to type those words, I knew that they would be okay together. I sobbed hysterically through every line not knowing how I'd make it to the next. Death had visited me more than enough times with them, and even if it didn't work out with Cody, I knew it was over. I finished composing my eternal love for them, cut the cords, and closed that chapter. My encounter with the Finch a few days earlier proved to be true.

The drive into town was a bittersweet one. I knew that I had to be content with my decision in letting them go. That way, I wouldn't bring that energy into my new doggy interview. It was a new page in a new chapter for me. So, I started it out by stopping at Ross to purchase some blankets, a new dog bed, collar, leash, and then to the grocery store for a few yummy treats. I had never rescued an animal from a shelter, much less been to one. I didn't know how any of it worked. I just wanted to make sure our meeting would be as natural and organic as possible.

There were health codes set in place to protect all involved, so they had me wait in the parking lot a bit longer than expected before I could go in and meet the little fellow. I actually had a few nerve balls playing dodgeball in my stomach as if I were on an audition at Paramount. Yet, once his lanky eight pounds walked into the room, they fizzled away like I had just booked the job. It was hilarious because, when he strolled in, he didn't run to me like all other dogs did in the previous three years. Instead, he lifted his leg and marked the side of the door. Then he took a few more steps before dropping a well-deserved dump from his extremely swollen anal glands. What a pleasant, "Hello to you, too," I thought. He finished taking his shelter shit and then became intrigued with everything in the room but me. It was obvious that the guy ruled the world and I was just a piece of matter there to distract him.

I knew I could play the game as well, so I pulled out my steak treats. In an instant, I was the only thing he was focused on. For the next fifteen minutes, we got to know each other even better. He was magnificent in every way, but I had to pee and felt it more appropriate to use the women's bathroom instead of marking the side of the door like he did. After hearing him bawl like a little baby all the way from the restroom, I knew it was a sealed deal. I came out and asked if that was him causing all the commotion, and it was. I buckled him into his new blue collar and leash, and we headed out to Forever Land!

As I was signing the papers, I asked if they knew anything about his background and how he made it to the shelter. They informed me that both he and his brother had been seen roaming through some nearby mountains for several weeks before finally being picked up by a good Samaritan. When the facility checked if both dogs were microchipped, they were. However, the owner declined in taking them back. Those are the pieces of shit you hate in the beginning, but then thank them for abandoning them so that someone more loving can take better care of them. I thought to myself, "How could anyone just ditch a dog in the wilderness to fend for himself, especially his size, and in the middle of winter?" No wonder he was a skinny little thing. Who knew how long they'd been out there trying to survive and how many of his siblings, if any, didn't make it?

I got to the last page of his adoption packet and was shocked when I read the medical report. The shelter had removed twelve of his teeth, all front and bottom, and a few others around his canines. He was only 3 years of awesome experience, had been neutered, and practically defanged. I was furious that any vet would remove that many teeth from a dog so young. I had always heard how "prescription happy" shelter vets were and how quickly they pulled teeth instead of trying to save them. What could we do right? We had to find a way to make the best of it, and I was proficient at it. Instead of doing it alone though, we now had each other to do it together.

We hopped into my SUV and I saw the fright in his eyes. In fact, it was turning him into *Benjamin Button*. He looked like a little old man drained with desperation. I picked him up out of his dog bed and placed him in my lap. His ears were glued to the back of his neck and his tears had stained his eyes so much that he looked like he'd been in a boxing match. I knew it would all change as soon as we got to our new home, took a bath, and slept on it for a few days. I also knew that he was no Cody. My little boy would become "Bodhi Moon."

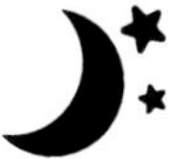

It had always amazed me how quickly a dog could get acclimated to a new territory. If only humans were the same. When we arrived back to the ranch, it was close to 9pm and both of us were exhausted. We pulled into the carport and Goldie went ballistics. Bodhi, a third of her size, wasn't a bit intimidated. I just wanted to make sure she didn't hurt him because she had no idea of her size and power. When Goldie played, she could knock down a 10-foot wall of cement blocks and nothing was going to stop her. She ran her usual 8,000 laps around half an acre of the property, while breaking the pathway lights, and layering her paws with mantles of mud. That was her form of introduction. When she was done, they sniffed butts and marked a few more yellow spots before getting out of the December snow.

There was a whole other arena inside that he also had to explore. As we headed in, I could see his big bright eyes light up with anticipation. Before checking the place out, he marked his territory right in front of the standing lamp to show us that he meant business. It was epic and would be the only time he'd ever sign his autograph inside again. After a few solid minutes surveying the rooms, I grabbed some shampoo and towels, and gave him a bath in the kitchen sink. He'd be further benefitted with luxurious amenities as if he was being pampered at a spa in Beverly Hills. It was obvious how much he appreciated being catered to.

We knew we made a fabulous decision. And, for the rest of the night, we would begin getting to know as much as we could of him. Two of his beds were positioned in different areas of the living room, and he had a third in my room. I decided to let him cuddle close to me on my own cushioned mattress since he was still pretty scared. It turned out to be a smart decision, because he had to get up two times to go outside and take a poop. If he hadn't been a foot away to alert me, that would've been a nice mess to clean up the next morning. His poor little shelter polluted stomach growled until the sun came up. But by that time, miraculously, he had returned back to looking like a little puppy. That would become a new chapter in my new book of my new love story!

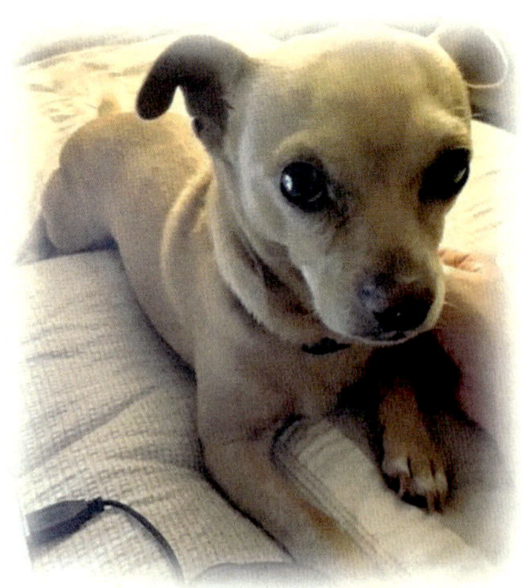

The holidays were upon us and, not but two days after bringing Bodhi into our world, we celebrated Christmas. We knew he was special, but had no idea the magnitude of nirvana he would bless our lives with. They say that Bodhi means "Enlightenment" and "Spiritual awakening." It would just so happen that one of the coolest spots in West Hollywood was "The Bodhi Tree Bookstore." I'd often stop by to browse the mystical works of art, info, events, and literature. Then I'd head down the way to grab an elixir at one of the herbal tea gardens and sit back, read my new book, and marinate in the Sanskrit world. That was always such a highlight for me because, on days when I felt the lowest of energies, I'd come out feeling calm as a muthr fkr. It was ethereal. Yet, it was absolutely real. That was Bodhi. Like all beloved dogs in my life, the messages from the celestials were in his eyes. His soul was filled with a constellation of stars. From the moon to the sun, the earth to the ocean, and everything in between... he was magical. I knew we were brought together into the entirely new cosmic vortex for a reason, and at the perfect time. He would turn out to be the best chance taken and the gift that would keep on giving.

Bodhi didn't have an alpha or type "A" personality bone in his body. He was a loving, gentle, observant, and extremely vibrant little super somebody. It was incredible to watch him come out of his shell just like the experiences I was blessed to share with Charly and Tippet. Just like them, he'd have his own sense of uniqueness.

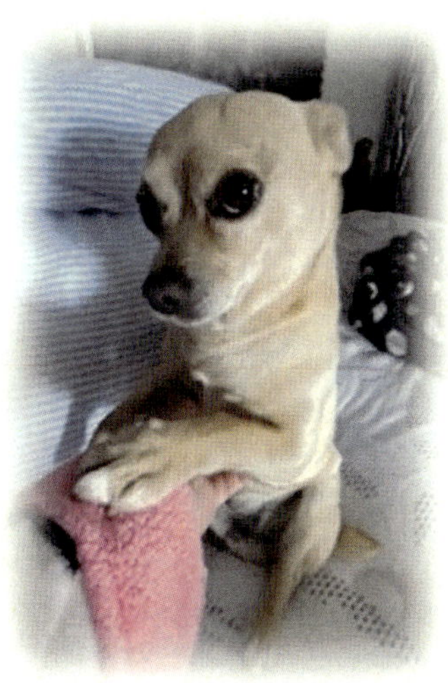

Within days, his anus shrank and he was sleeping deeply through the night. His butt was still sensitive so we took extra care when picking him up. We switched his diet to a softer nutritious format to accommodate his lack of teeth. Yet, we still gave him homemade bones to strengthen the ones he had left. He played with sticks, chased Goldie, and took time sitting in the sun soaking up the winter rays. Then on snow days, he'd tiptoe through the blizzard needing you to hold his paw like a toddler. There was no end to his curiosity and the chilly weather didn't stop him from absorbing everything.

As we'd have dinner at my stepdad's, Bodhi would also get to know his dogs, "Dasey" and "Selina." They were gentle loving seniors with demeanors as soft as sheer snowflakes. They instantly loved him. His third canine was a giant sweetheart as well. But when he took him in as a stray twelve years earlier, he was a fighter. "Huevos" was separated in an outside enclosure to keep him from escaping, but we didn't know if he'd attack Bodhi. I certainly kept Bodhi away from the feral cat, "Estrella." She was a love bug, but ate rabbits his size. I didn't want his foot to become the lucky charm on my car mirror.

Unfortunately, Dasey was on her last leg. Her mom, Lucky, had passed away a year earlier from a stroke that she never recovered from. They were deeply bonded. So, when Dasey lost her mama, she began to go downhill. Her quality of life had reached a point where my stepdad knew that he had to put her down. It was sad to watch him struggle weekly with changing his mind. She was his precious little girl and another one of the loves of his life. The timing of death would never come easy as it reminded him of losing his soulmate three years earlier. Spike had been his best friend for nineteen amazing years, and now Dasey (far left) would join him and her mom.

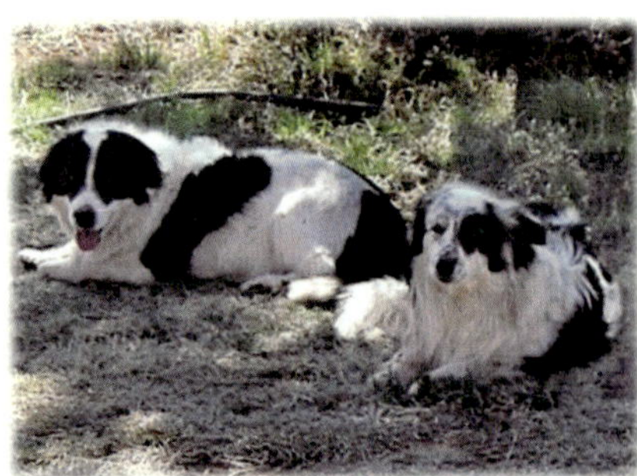

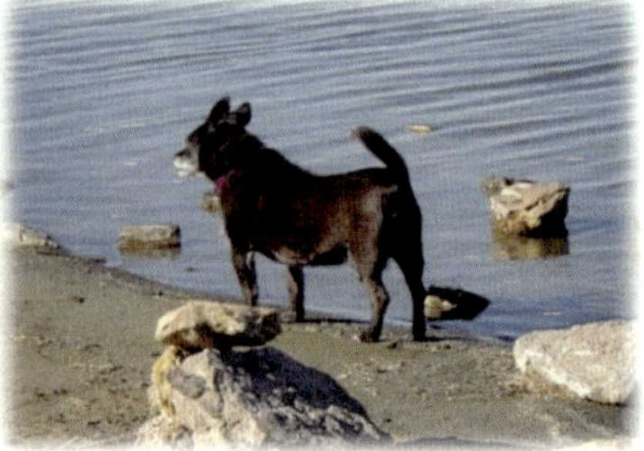

I felt as if Bodhi was an intricate part of all of our rebirths. He arrived just as Dasey was about to transition from one form to another. Beautifully, he was able to meet her, assimilate her energy, and circulate the succession of her legacy. What a special sendoff to the new destination awaiting her. The sadness Dasey's death would bring to us all was, in a way, healthily overshadowed by the new youthful energy of Bodhi. How could you not love him and not love to be around him? There was no way he'd let you sulk in sorrow. He knew you had to heal. He just knew how to comfort you along the way. From that time forward, he'd always have a special type of warmth in my mom and stepdad's hearts.

Upon Dasey's passing, we had found a veterinarian who had helped make the experience as comforting as possible. So, I decided to take Bodhi into the office for his first checkup. Of course, everyone fell in love with him. Other than not wanting anyone near his ass, we were able to walk out with a clean bill of health.

He started responding quickly to words, commands, tones, and energy, and even learned how to shake hands thanks to Goldie. Yet, it took him a minute to get used to his name. I found it hard to believe since it sounded so similar to his previous one. I began to realize that he was just playing me. Bodhi was extremely intelligent and it was his way of showing me that he only listened when he wanted to.

He didn't bark or give any licks right away, and would pull back if I tried to kiss his face. That would change after being gone and out of sight for more than ten minutes. We could hear him howl from the next house over. When I'd pull into the ranch, he'd race out the door, jump into my arms, and try his best to slobber me with wet kisses. The only thing was that Bodhi was green in that category. He would crash into my face without knowing which area to kiss, or how to kiss, just like an inexperienced 7th grader smooches his first girlfriend. I thought, at times, he was going to poke my eye out. It was adorable, and the beginning to so many of our winning moments together.

He had become attached to me, but still wouldn't let me anywhere near his butt. I began to relate it to his Root chakra since he had been dumped by his previous owners and, more than likely, lost his sense of grounding and security. It was comical in the beginning, but I realized that it probably had something to do with how he ended up with half a tail. When I met him, I noticed that a decent portion of it had been chopped off. I didn't want to imagine what other abuse he might have endured, as I sensed it wasn't a happy experience for him. We took the issue seriously and had no problem working through his discomfort until he was ready to talk about it. Our main goal was to provide him with all the love, comfort, protection, food, fun, health, and trust as possible. Once he could get rooted again, we knew he would excel.

I began to see similar traits to those of Charly and Tippet. He'd run on three legs, kick dirt up after he peed, lay on the bathroom rug (or on my dirty clothes) while I took a shower, and would race around the house after getting a bath. He immediately learned words like, "You wanna go outside?" – "Let's go pee" – "You're such a good boy" – and eagerly picked up on, "Are you hungry?" He also related to the nicknames, "Bobes" – "Bodes" – "Bobo" – "Bobee" – and "Sweet Pea." And without a doubt, he understood, "I love you."

Bodhi also saw ghosts and spirits just like Tippet did. I remember my ex undermining Tip's ability to ward off unwanted energies. Then a translucent figure, resembling his late brother, showed up on our security cameras. He never admitted to Tippet's special powers, even after instances where pictures mysteriously fell off the walls upstairs. We'd find broken glass everywhere. Bodhi must've inherited those peculiar features, because I'd catch him suddenly squeal and jump out of his skeleton when the paranormal beings came to greet him.

Although he had secured his spot next to me in bed, he also had his favorite blankie just like Charly did. Interestingly, he gravitated to the simple gray covering. I could sense early on that he was a living, breathing instrument that would signify the Helpful People and Travel section of a Feng Shui Bagua. He'd sit next to me while typing in my journal, meditate with me in silence, and cuddle his little head on my pillow while we both headed into dreamland listening to Solfeggios. He was my road dog and went with me everywhere. When he wasn't holding my hand with his paw, he would stick his head out of the window to breathe in the fresh mountain air. On days when the drive was longer than usual, he'd rest his head in my hand and take a nap.

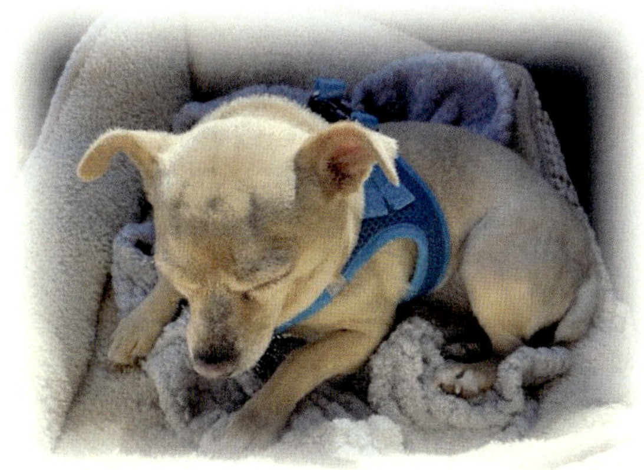

"Good morning" was always my signature greeting. And as with Charly and Tippet, it brightened every moment no matter what part of the day it was. Some of our favorite times would begin at sunrise when I'd wake up seeing his beautiful brown lenses and tender expression telling me, *"Let's get up and have another wonderful experience."* He'd take a huge stretch, lay on his back, and have me rub his chest and belly for another five minutes. Then I'd cup his mouth and cold, moist nose with my hand, and rub all around his cheeks and chin. That was his trademark move for affection. I'd conclude the doting ritual by rubbing his Third Eye to help expand his dynamic power of intuition and higher light.

Bodhi would get so lively in those moments that I'd see his walls breaking down and his trust building back up. I'd savor in those am hours, primarily because it kept Goldie at bay and allowed us to enjoy some one-on-one time together. It also gave him the chance to play with his favorite toy: *The Little Donut*. That cushioned pink pastry went everywhere with us. He'd play with it, chew it up, and then sleep on it whenever he needed some zzzz's. It reminded me of *Little Duckie* and how much fun Charly and Tippet had with him. Although Bodhi couldn't jump up on the bed, he didn't have any problem leaping off. He'd follow me into every room, lay on me while I stretched and did sit-ups, and stayed by my side through every footstep. I'd even bring him to my mom's office on weekends so that I could make some money. He'd have fun. But, when he was done, he was done.

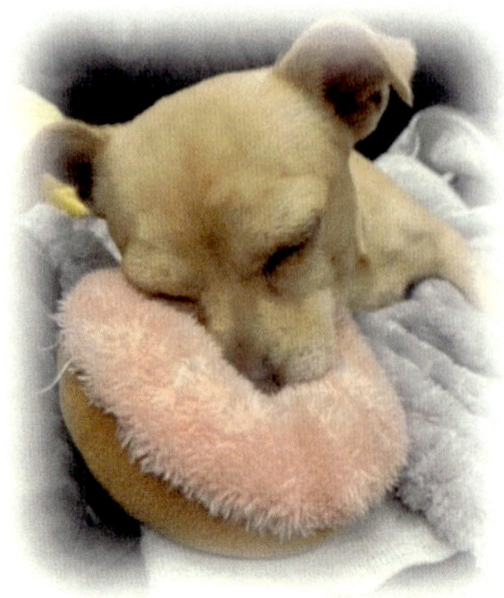

It was true love at first site for Bodhi and me. The immediate closeness of our bond began in that little room and would carry on into future lifetimes. I could tell that we were in for an amazing ride together. I didn't know how anyone could survive being dropped off in an unfamiliar place, by those you trusted most, only for them not to ever come back for you. Then, you end up in a prison.

It was likely that Bodhi was going to have some kind of PTSD stored somewhere, but he was a fighter. He was a little bundle of gluten-free bread who had made it through the wilderness and in the middle of winter. Nothing was going to stop him from living the best life ever. I knew he'd have some attachment and anxiety issues, and I knew it was going to take some time. I also knew that we were soulmates. That meant I was going to help him relearn and regain his trust in humans. No matter how long or how much work it would take, I was going to help get him to a place where he could live happily and freely.

I was well aware that Bodhi didn't need me to survive the basics of life. But in those first few months, I had to provide him with enough of a sturdy foundation that he could eventually take on his own world much more independently. Isn't that what we all want for our kids? Only, the difference between a pet and a child is that our dog doesn't graduate from high school, go on to college, travel overseas, move in with friends, get married, or venture in and out of jobs until they find their true calling. They need us a 100% for their entire lives.

I had seen Charly and Tippet blossom and it was one of the most beautiful things to be a part of. It was going to be just as amazing to watch Bodhi do the same. I knew that Charly and Tippet's spirits would channel through him, so I'd be able to energetically engage with them through his choices and movements. How lucky was I to be able to carry on with their stories?

Since Bodhi appeared in my life, my nightmares began to fade away and I was finally able to get a good eight hours of sleep like I used to. I'm sure diffusing essential oils throughout my room, EFT tapping, meditating, and journaling also contributed to the triumph. But Bodhi was the culprit. Things were looking much brighter for the first time in four months.

I began to see him as a furry Tree of Life who kept all branches lovingly fused together with a transformational glow. Without question, he was on point with inner wellness being the source of outer happiness. His fresh energy was so positively contagious that even my plants began returning to their pizazz. They, too, were devastated upon our eviction. In fact, I lost most of them. The ones that survived did so with the last bit of saved hydration that had hibernated in their mangled roots. They had been repotted and re-soiled. But because of Bodhi, they reconnected back with their souls. Revival and restoration were upon us all!

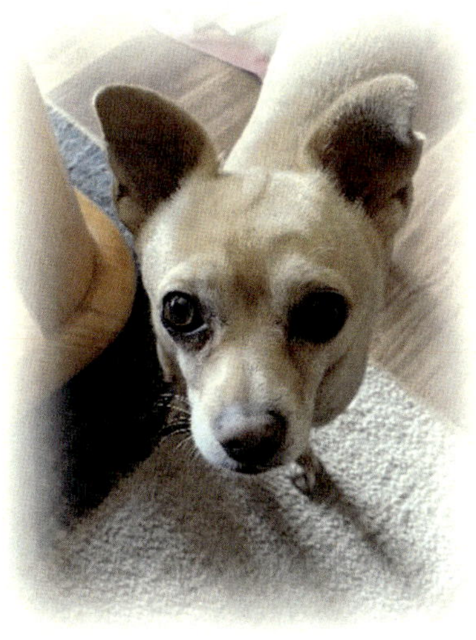

I remembered when I lived in LA and not ever understanding how my neighbors would baby talk to their infants and kids and grandkids the way they did.

"Hi boo boo gaga – *(kissy sounds)* – my little sweet pea – look at my precious baby – yes you are, my honey bear babas – you're such a good girl – *(clapping)* – did you go poopies – yes you did, stinkers – I hear your tummies – oh my goodness, my little princess – look at those teethies – I'm gonna give you kissies *(kissy sounds)* – and hugsies – *(love squeezes)* – and never let go of you, my baby..."

Then I adopted Bodhi.

I had begun the lingo with Charly and Tippet over three years earlier and remembered people looking at me like I was out of my freaken mind for talking to them in those tones. Bodhi brought it back to the forefront as it was official: I WAS A SINGLE PET PARENT!!!

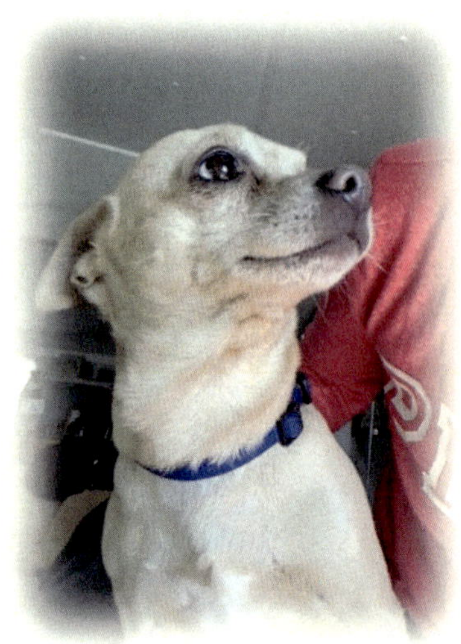

7
Lola and the Little Dipper

Three months had passed and the joy that Bodhi brought to our lives was incredible. He was such a little angel and my cosmic soul child. He had gained over three pounds, started barking, howling, and licking faces. He also became a serial tail wagger. It was truly amazing how much he was shifting in form. Even his front bowed leg appeared to have straightened. In the time he'd been sharing energy with us, I had become active and mobile again, and even with a bit of dedication. I was working out in baby steps, writing, being social, and posting on my public pages. I also dove back into some of my creative work as well as ideas for businesses I wanted to start someday. Luckily, my mom talked me into returning to acupuncture. Before I knew it, I was enjoying some humor.

I had been on a handful of local auditions in the three years I was in my relationship, and another few in the time I was living with my parents. Yet, I didn't get a single callback or booking. I put in my prep work and performed great on each, but just wasn't what they were looking for. Productions were coming to the state in massive numbers, but the roles were limited. LA actors led those projects while the locals had to fight for the small leftover parts.

As grateful as I was for being called in to audition, I felt like I was going backwards. In no way had I evolved anywhere close to being a powerhouse player who could choose their roles. I hadn't even worked a steady paying entertainment job in eleven years. Who was I to complain? But I had started my career in the mecca of the showbiz capital and now I was competing with an entire state for one liners and extra work. Other than the two breakout roles I was called in for, there was nothing about those job interviews that were rewarding, or that inspired me to want to continue acting. I think I just felt that it was all I had left. It was all I had ever done, and so the fear of having to do something else sunk in.

Then came *Furever Soulmates*. I had been learning and growing with Bodhi, and was fascinated with his progress and transition from being abandoned to getting rescued. My interest in helping other doggies began expanding. I was intrigued on how the powers of love and comfort could bring an animal back to life and vice versa for their accommodating humans. My initial goal was to expand the awareness of pet adoption: ***"Adopt a pet, gain a soulmate!"*** It was that easy and that real! I wanted to do all I could in connecting shelter animals with safe, loving, forever homes. Every day, I'd extend my search to areas throughout the state, the metro city, and even the borderline communities for all animals in need. Then I'd post them on my social media pages in hopes that they'd cross someone who was interested.

I didn't have a clue what was in store for me, but I had the compassion and desire to get homeless, unwanted, hospice, abused, and forgotten pets the affection they deserved. The soul-searching space that my parents offered me, in hopes of helping me fly again, was helping me to help deprived animals to do the same. I had Bodhi, and we were writing the perfect start to another perfect story!

I didn't know if I had anything to do with the pets I posted getting adopted, but it sure was gratifying seeing how many of those animals got connected with their forever companions. I always said that, "It only takes one." Maybe that one person ran across that one posting, shared it with one other, and landed on the laptop of the one perfect somebody. Who knew? I did, however, feel that fate was calling me.

Before long, I began shifting my original goal into something even more meaningful. I kept coming across an overflow of seniors that had been dumped at shelters, picked up as strays, or found in horrific hoarding cases. I used the word "dump" because a discarder didn't merit the privilege of using the term "surrender" in regard to any animal. When someone gives up on their pet, they don't surrender them; they abandon them. It's especially devastating when that pet is sick, disabled, had been sick for some time, and the owner allowed them to suffer long term before ditching them. If they couldn't have the decency, empathy, and consideration to make the proper arrangements for those darling souls to be taken care of in their absence, illness, or selfishness, then I had zero respect for them.

People's health fails, they get old, and pass away. They lose jobs, move, have kids, and want to travel more. Their circumstances change, they can't afford meds, or can't watch their pets die. Rarely is it understandable for a family member to be ditched at a shelter; high-kill nonetheless. Even worse, is leaving them chained up in the yards they moved from. Pets deserve to have something safer set up for them ahead of time. They deserve to smoothly go into another home with someone who could tend to their needs and have the strength to stick it out to the end. How dare people remove those darlings from the only place they've ever known, and throw them out like trash. That's what happens when laws deem pets as property. When people don't have use for them anymore, they toss them. I've never had any leniency for those who neglect a pet in any way ever since doing it myself as a kid, and living with that guilt as an adult.

My newfound undertaking then became, *"**There are no age limits on Soulmates.**"* My focus was on seniors and those with special needs. I had to get as many as I could out of the shelters and into ideal homes where they'd live out their best lives. I just wanted to save them all. But since that wasn't a reality for me at the time, I had to find other ways. Bodhi had motivated me to do that for all the elderly treasures out there. Just like that fateful day when his charming face grazed my page, another life-changing 4-pawed being found me.

I came across his magnetic energy one day when I was doing a quick search on newly available animals throughout the state. He was in the form of an 18 ½-year creamy white sensational little Chihuahua with melt-worthy eyes and an adorable face. He had been turned in at a facility in the metro city. If ever I felt sickened by anything done to an animal in the past, that was it. The poor baby had been placed in a cage and left to die in the shelter all alone.

I wasn't in a position to adopt another dog, nor was that my intent. I just wanted to get him out of there. I monitored him daily for a week just praying that a good Samaritan would offer him the comfort of a caring, secure, peaceful place to live out his final days. Unfortunately, he was still there. I was so saddened to see that nobody had stepped up to the plate. It was then that I decided to take an even bigger chance than I did with Bodhi. He was coming home with me!

It was a Thursday that I'll never forget. The shelter didn't know much about him other than being housed in the medical unit due to kennel cough. When I asked if anyone else had come to visit, they said, "No, he's 18 years old." I sat on the floor awaiting his presence, not having any idea what I was about to get myself into. By the way they spoke of him, you would've thought he was on his deathbed. I was just hoping that he'd be strong enough to walk. When he entered the room, I knew he was the one.

His name was "Dipper" and his fur was a pink hue, which was apparent of an infection. He was frail, disheveled, and dirty. His spine was curved like a hunchbacked old man with part of his lumbar vertebrae protruding out. He had solid crusties glued to the inner creases of his eyes and the skin under his chin was raw. He barely had any hair on his ears and they were lined with black scabies. He was hacking profusely, but when I put out my hands to pet him, he walked over and fell into them. It was awful to see that little boy in such horrible shape. I wanted to cry, but pulled out a steak treat instead. For a moment, he was able to forget how painful everything was. I never wanted to leave him, but I couldn't take a chance with Bodhi getting infected. I had to go back to the ranch to prepare him for the arrival of his new brother. Interestingly, I wasn't worried that my mom would say, "No." There was something that sure of him. I had a week to get the place ready for his welcoming home party!

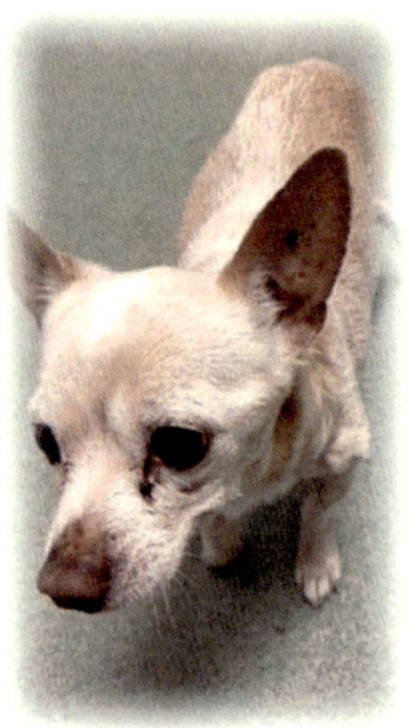
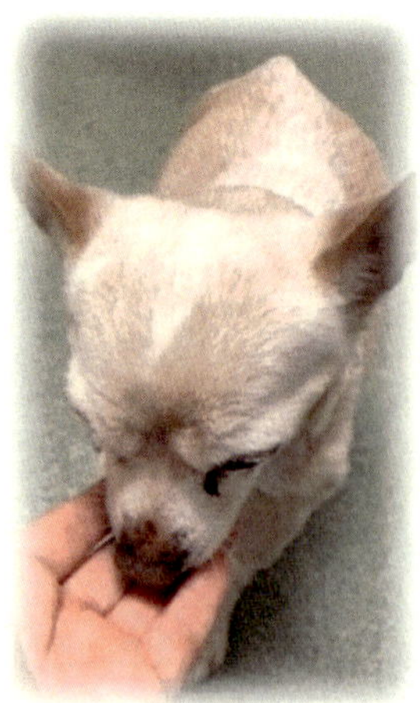
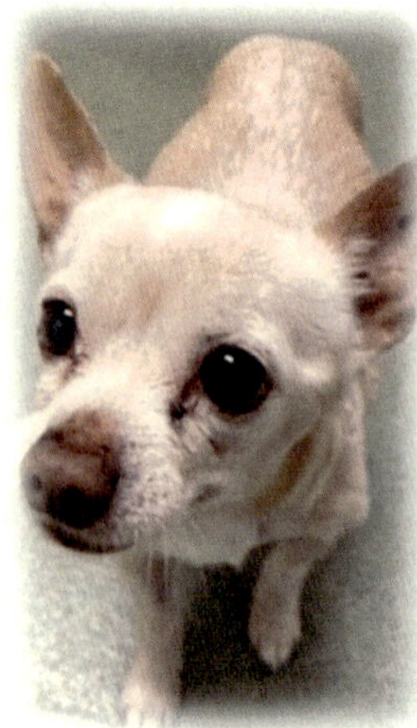

From the moment I laid eyes on him, I never took my mind or attention off of him. It was pure love at first sight... again. Although my intent was to get him out of that facility so that he wouldn't die in there, I would be gifted with so much more!

In the six days we were waiting for the little guy to get better, I made the arrangements to bring even another doggy into our lives. I know right? I wasn't in any position to adopt one dog and now I was setting up my third. Yikes!!! She was also a senior, 12 years of age, and had been handed over to a shelter in the southern part of the state. I was told that her owner developed dementia and began abusing her. She was brought in by the woman's adult children who notified the workers that the dog was being kicked and hung by her own leash. She was much smaller than Bodhi, and a tiny little purebred cream-colored Chihuahua with adorable bubbly eyes and the impression of intimidation. Like my future 18 ½-year companion, something told me that I could save her.

Bodhi loved playing outside with Goldie and Goldie enjoyed it just as much. They had developed a formula where she would allow him to bite the side of her face with what teeth he had left as if he was the bigger and stronger dog. As cute as it was, Goldie had begun picking on him and playing with him way too roughly. He never protested, but I noticed the uneasiness and didn't like it one bit. I didn't want her intrusive behavior to switch up his playful personality into anything timid, cowardly, or even mean. Bodhi wasn't a dog that needed to be in charge or dominant in any way. He was the farthest from it and that atmosphere was nowhere in his nature. But she was ruining the adventure.

Goldie would steal his toys, bones, and his beds even though her 50-pound body couldn't fit in them. Every time he wanted to play with me, she made it impossible. She was becoming a pest and Bodhi was getting deprived. Then her bratty, selfish behavior got even worse as my parents enabled her. She would roll around in the weeds and dirt all day, throw up in the house, eat grasshoppers and Chincharas, and then they'd let her run around inside the place just as rambunctious. On top of that, they'd have no problem with her jumping on the couch while we were eating, and all over the guests who came to visit.

I purged the house daily so that every piece of furniture wouldn't be lathered with hair, dust, and stinky dog smell. Not only did Goldie bring in dirt, but she had digestive and flatulence issues. Every night, my hard work went to waste. They didn't babysit her all day like I did. They didn't pick up her vomit and diarrhea. Plus, they left it up to me to feed her. I was stuck and irritated, grossed out and exhausted, and my parents were just adding to it. I understood that I was in their home and she was a dog they loved just like I did Bodhi. So, I had to suck it up and respect it. Yet, my temperament went from being nice and loving to being annoyed with her. We definitely became divided.

One of the main reasons I considered a third dog was to save her, but to also help Bodhi prosper like a 3-year-old dog should. Goldie was turning into a spoiled brat and I knew his future older brother would take more of my time and attention. Maybe getting him a friend, his size, would help him develop into the amazing young dog he was developing into. As much as I wanted, I couldn't take him with me everywhere. Since he still hadn't fully shed his attachment issues, I wanted to ease his worries. I thought she might help take his mind off me when I was gone, instead of being home by himself.

That weekend, I talked my mom into driving the four hours to see the 12-year-young princess. The shelter wasn't really a shelter, but more like a temporary housing unit where animals were dropped off, adopted, and shipped off. I didn't see any medical professionals on site, but maybe that was a good thing. That area of the state lacked funding for shelters, so bless their hearts for doing the best that they could. The staff members were absolutely amazing.

Her name was "Lola" and when they brought her out, she was even tinier than expected. She didn't take to me right away, but it was understandable. Bodhi peed and took a dump upon our introduction, so how was I to expect anything different? I asked if she got along with other dogs and they said that she was great with other dogs. I took their word for it and went to get Bodhi. His loving self trotted right in and she immediately attacked him. That didn't sit well with me. I thought maybe I had made a huge mistake in contemplating another dog, especially that one. The staff reassured me that she was surprisingly acting different. Long story short, I went against my gut.

She seemed to know her name, so I kept it and added Moon just like I did with Bodhi. From that moment on, we began an interesting journey with our 2nd planetary sphere in the form of a 6-pound furball named, "Miss Lola Moon."

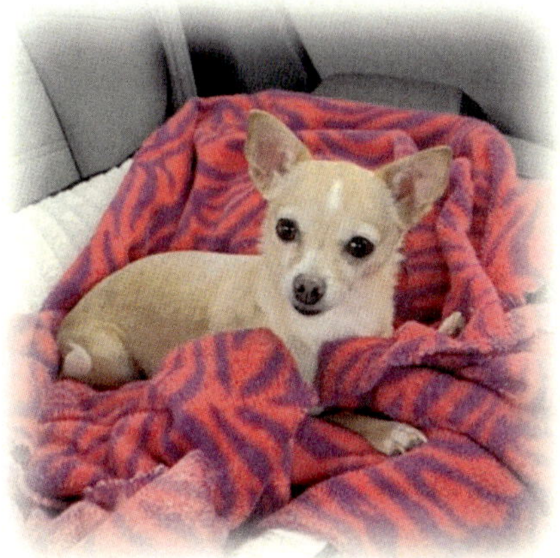

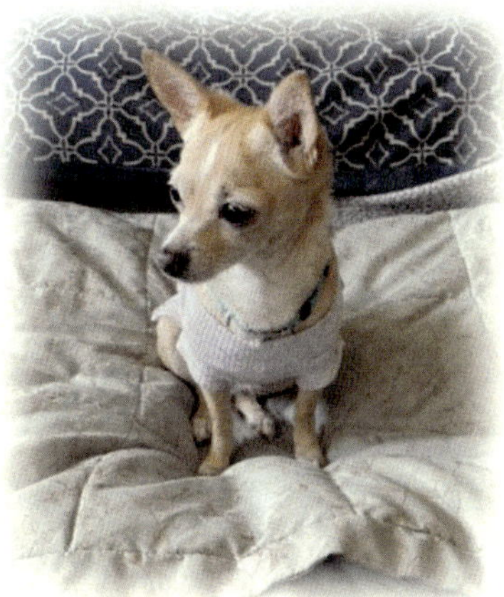

In the next few days, we noticed that she was a spunky little creature and seemed to be closer to 2 years of age rather than 12. She owned a mouthful of piranha teeth with some seriously bad breath, and was clearly missing a screw on the friendly board. She was mean, territorial, aggressive, and exhibited an "A" type of personality to the max. I didn't like it and was extremely disappointed. Regret began sinking in because none of our animal family members represented that kind of presence. We quickly found out that she wasn't spayed, but the blame was on me for not checking her medical and health history before adopting. Poor Bodhi was in fear on a constant basis. One minute she'd want to play with him; the next she wanted to kill him. I wasn't resonating with her at all.

Not but three days later, we headed back to the metro city to pick up Dipper. It was day 16, which had always been a lucky number for me. I was hoping it would be a lucky number for my new soulmate as well. When I walked into the shelter to get him, the volunteer acted like it was a burden. He grunted as we headed to the room. Upon entering, he told me that he didn't want to have to disinfect the whole space when we were done, so he was just going to place him on the table. Then he walked off. What a not so pleasant way to start the experience. He returned with Dipper in his arms, placed him on the exam counter, and said, "Here's the grumpy old man." I would've probably given him a mouthful, but I kept my energy on my new little boy. We were already winning by getting him out of that place.

Our second meeting was even more enchanting than our first. He wasn't as pink anymore, so I knew he was doing better. He was still coughing, but not nearly as bad or as deep. I did, however, notice that he was deaf. I snapped my fingers and clapped my hands, and Dip didn't budge. The guy tried to tell me otherwise, but I already knew that he didn't know anything about my dog. Dipper was deaf and it didn't make a difference; I was still adopting him. The guy took him away while I went up to the front to get his paperwork.

As I was reading through his medical history, I noticed a slew of reported ailments. He was listed as Geriatric, had mild anemia, mild neutrophilia, mild monocytosis, and congestive heart failure with a 4/6 grade heart murmur. The notes indicated a swollen abdomen, kyphosis (curved spine), five teeth extracted from an already twelve missing, was on antibiotics and bronchitis medication, and had been given three vaccinations (including Rabies and Distemper). He had also been neutered by the shelter. I WAS FURIOUS!!! Who neuters and pumps so much medication into an 18 ½-year-old dog? Who would put a dog that age through that kind of trauma, and on anesthesia? He had already suffered enough emotional anguish for a vet to unnecessarily clip his balls. It wasn't like he was humping around; he could barely walk. I had been learning about the state's spay/neuter laws, the downside of shelters, and the types of policies they operated by ever since adopting Bodhi. But that was ridiculous.

On top of that, he was free of charge. I thought, "No way, he's worth so much more." I handed the worker a hundred-dollar bill and signed the last of his papers. I was pissed and just wanted to get him out of that building. Nobody came and took our picture. Nobody came to say goodbye to him. Nobody paid an ounce of attention. The energy that day at the shelter set the stage for how much more I would give to that dog while he was still here on this earth. I wrapped him up in his blankie, took a selfie, and got us out of there.

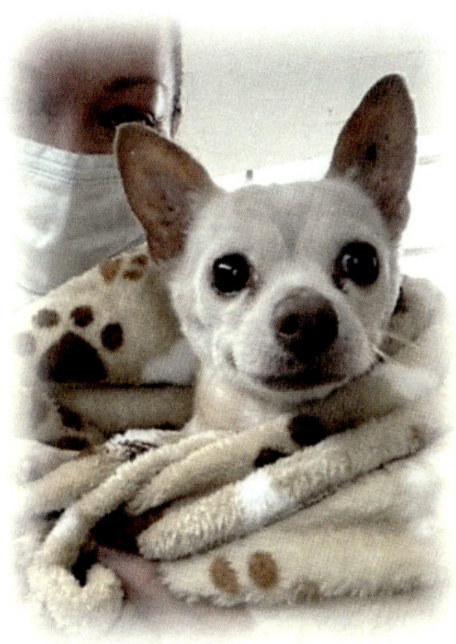

The eagerness in his eyes was something I couldn't explain. Not but a few feet from walking out of the shelter, I put him down for just a few minutes to pee. Instead, he began racing in the opposite direction as if trying to escape. For a dog who could barely move in that room an hour earlier, he wasn't showing an ounce of being disabled. He was still disoriented and couldn't figure out which way to go, but I could tell that he felt so free! I let him wander around a bit more so that he could let out the last of that place's energy that was stuck inside of his bladder and large intestine.

I finally loaded him in one of his new beds in the front seat. Bodhi and Lola were chilled in the back and didn't know how to react. My stepbrother had been staying with them while I was inside taking care of business. The cold dark clouds were stirring up as a sign for us to exit the premises. We didn't make it to the first light before I noticed that Dip couldn't sit still. I knew he was frightened and filled with uncertainty. I couldn't imagine how every chemical was twisting the insides of his body. I pulled over and placed him on my lap for the rest of the drive home. That would be the first of a lifetime of trips for us.

When we arrived, I was a bit reluctant to let him walk around, primarily because of Goldie. He wasn't in the shape to be rolled in the dirt. Once I took him out of my vehicle, he surprisingly began to explore like a normal dog. I was in awe! He was sniffing and marking and trotting slowly through the property. Then asshole Lola attacked him. She launched her teeth into his neck and pinned him onto the ground. I about lost my sanity. Poor little Dip got up limping and perplexed, and with dirt smudged all over his eyebrows. He tried his best to walk it off, but I immediately ran over to pick him up. His skeleton was so delicate that I could hear his bones crack when I lifted his torso. The assault didn't seem to bother him as much as it bothered me. After a few kisses and hugs, I put him back down. Not but two minutes later, Bodhi shockingly did the same thing!!! OMG!!! I was beside myself!!! I smacked his little ass and almost sent him to Uranus! Then I picked up Dip so that nobody could come close to him again. The frightful look on his bewildered face broke my heart. From that moment on, I knew that him and I would be inseparable.

We went inside and the first thing he did was sniff the place out. Bodhi and Lola were on my shitlist, so I had my mom keep them at bay. He seemed interested, but meticulously took his time investigating the rooms. After he made his rounds, I filled up the kitchen sink and gave him a bath just like both of my other rescues. I gently scrubbed the solid crusty off of his eye and got the shelter smell off of his fur. He didn't fight me at all. It was kind of like he was just waiting for the trauma to be cleansed away. The experience was so spiritually purifying for the both of us.

I dried him off, put on one of his new little green Heart chakra hoodies, and offered him some delicious soft shredded chicken and broth. He was starving and exhausted, and devoured the food. Then, we put him on the couch to pass out. It was evident that he was never going to be able to jump high enough on anything over five or six inches, jump down from anything the same height, or be able to walk up any stairs. That was alright. He only weighed eight illustrious pounds. It would never be a bother to help him travel.

Dipper was the third of our planetary orbs and the projected number of the highest power. The number "3" always had a unique significance in my spiritual world. I thought it to be a symbol of harmony, wisdom, and understanding, and that which characterized time: past, present, future – birth, life, death – beginning, middle, end. It represented "The Divine." I hadn't planned it that way, but that's how it crystalized. I was always drawn to "3" since I was a kid, whether it be my uniform label, to the grouping of lessons that came to me, to inspirations, manifestations, blessings, or deaths. Directly or indirectly, that number was a part of who I was. Dipper had landed the spot of our 3rd Moon and, by far, the most galactic.

After that initial meeting, Bodhi never attacked him again. I think he was just peer pressured by Lola, or he was trying to be a badass and impress her like immature dudes do. The concept faded and he, Lola, and Dipper ended up napping close together on the couch for a few more hours. My parents and I relaxed and had dinner.

When it was time to call it a night, I picked up Dip's fragile little body and carried him into my bedroom to get him situated in one of the three cushioned doggy beds awaiting him on the floor. I couldn't take a chance with putting him on my bed because I didn't want him to fall off when I was deep in sleep slobber. I gently hugged him and rubbed my nose on the side of his face while I wished him a beautiful night's sleep. Then I looked into his sweet little eyes and told him that I loved him. He softened into the comfort of his blankies and slowly fell into dreamland. I plopped Bodhi next to my pillow and Lola a bit lower, and then shut off the lights. Our first evening together was a success and the rest of the midnight hours would be the beginning to the most amazing story of my life. Welcome Home "Dipper Moon!!!"

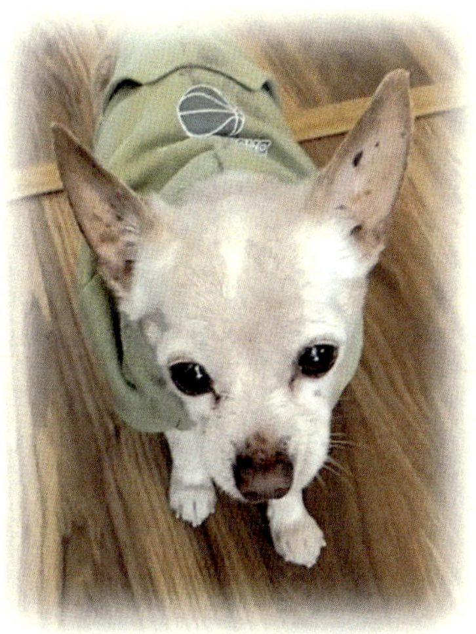

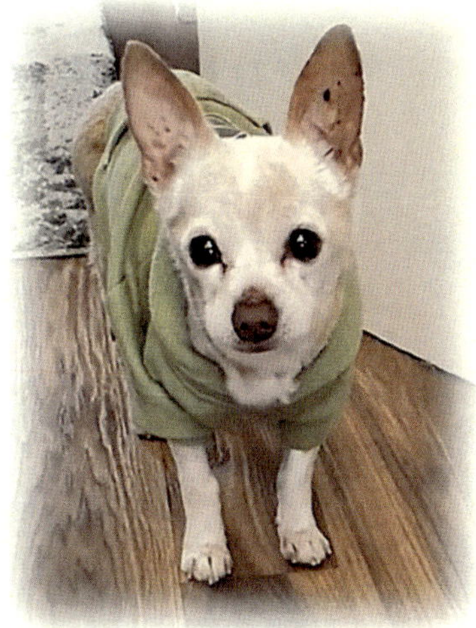

Early that next morning, I got up and took Dip outside for his first real walk. He could barely maneuver his legs and balance at that time. It was much different than his exit from the shelter. It was as if he did all he could to keep himself upright and standing the previous day, that he couldn't help but be depleted. I could tell that he knew he was safe and protected. He just had that sparkle throughout his entire aura. Physically, though, he had a few rough patches we'd have to work on. His little butt was extremely swollen just like Bodhi's was, the arch in his back was protruding, his empty scrotum was nearly touching the ground, and he had a difficult time breathing. He just couldn't inhale without strain and the sound of built-up phlegm.

Once he got a little air and exercise, I took him back inside to treat him to another nutritious homemade specialty. He devoured it once again, then went into his room to sleep it off. Since I was present, him and I laid on top of my bedspread and fleece blanket. I'll never forget how innocent and purely magical he looked as he settled his anatomy into the comfy covers. His new turtleneck sweater kept him warm and cozy, and the diffused vetiver and frankincense essential oils added a touch of tranquility. I ran my hands across the back of his torso and just watched him enjoy his moment. He was smiling the entire time he was sleeping. I had never seen a dog do that before. That would become one of his famous trademarks. I knew he was going to change my life as I loved him instantly. It was like he was my new baby, my new little boy, and I was going to do whatever it took to make sure his remaining time on this marble would be the best time he ever had.

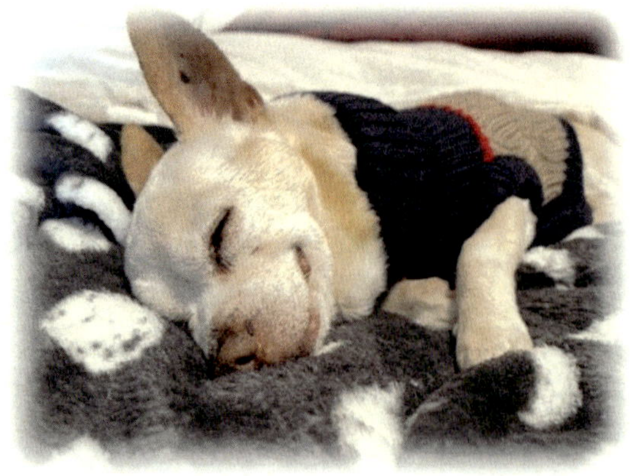

Later in the afternoon, I took him to his first acupuncture and laser therapy treatment. What a great sport he was. He stood there calm and mellow while she poked him with needles. If there was a sensitive spot, he'd twitch for a second, but then bury his head in my lap while I rubbed him. He never yelped once. The alternative practitioner thought that it was likely he had arthritis, but nothing was listed anywhere on his paperwork. Therefore, we had to monitor him and see how he reacted to the treatment. I knew it was going to do wonders for his life because acupuncture had saved mine.

The next day, I took him to get his blood work and first checkup. The medical veterinarian believed that Dip had an enlarged heart and collapsed trachea. She wasn't able to take x-rays because Dip wasn't having any of it. He had just spent two weeks caged in the shelter's medical unit. The doctor had to speculate based on her examination and how he reacted from placing pressure on his throat and chest. Like Bodhi, we walked out of that office with a positive outlook.

Before we took off, I went through his reports again while in the parking lot. I noticed that he didn't have the cough upon entering the shelter. He actually developed the hacking after the dental surgery and castration. I understood the benefits of his teeth being removed, but it seemed that the tube they inserted into his throat for anesthesia most likely caused his trachea to collapse. Who knew? I wasn't a veterinarian. Yet, something shifted after those procedures. And now, Dip was going to suffer with throat discomfort for the rest of his life. What a shame. All we could do was continue trying to make things better in the ways we could. I decided that one of those ways would be to pick up a top-of-the line HEPA purifier before heading back home to help ensure fresh air for his respiratory system. The clearer his throat and lungs were, the better. I was going to do all I could to make sure that he breathed as painless as possible.

After just one day, my little boy was a whole different dog. He was running and trotting and only showed little signs of joint pain. We quickly began learning how to naturally accommodate him. Because of his age and gravity, his gums had sunk into the sides of his cheeks and overlapped his teeth. He couldn't really get a grip on solid food. He had several choppers left and would eventually show us how sharp they were when snatching food from our hands. I just wanted to give him the convenience of ground-up meals in the meantime. I also didn't want to give any of my dogs processed kibble or canned food. They all got organic meat, vitamins, and steamed organic vegetables twice a day. Dipper's metabolism was much faster, so he'd get three meals. His breath was a bit harsh in the beginning just like Lola's. But that would fade with the addition of better nutrition. He also drank water constantly, so that helped tremendously.

Dipper was definitely a pee'er and usually on the hour. That was a good thing, because the vet informed me that fluid had the possibility of building up in his lungs with heart disease. She wanted to prescribe him a diuretic, but I was already ahead of her in a more natural, homeopathic way. Since having Bodhi, I had started learning more about the non-medicinal remedies and treatments for dogs. I had always been on the same path as a human and wanted to provide that gentle care to my pets for optimal health as well. I wanted to help build the functions of their own immune systems so that they could fight illness and disease as naturally as they could. By the time I brought Dipper into my life, I had ordered him non-synthetic herbs, vitamins, and tonics for his heart. Along with weekly acupuncture and laser therapy, he began flourishing... and quickly!!! I could also tell that the anesthesia, antibiotics, and rest of the medication that the shelter had polluted him with were flushing out of his system.

Dipper had the cutest little paws. But for some reason, he had no traction. He most likely was an indoor dog, but you would've never known after seeing him probe the property. At the time he entered our lives, my mom's place was furnished with hardwood flooring. Within weeks, we filled those areas in with rugs so that he wouldn't slip every time he took a step. Within months, the entire place was covered with soft wool runners as if he was walking on carpet. Since the alternative doctor met us at my mom's office very week for his treatments, he would take full advantage of actual carpet. Then we'd head outside to finish it off with a walk, and he'd turn into a superhero on the cement. It was interesting because he didn't seem to have a problem walking on the mixed gravel pathway on the property. Down the road, he'd even run on it. I could tell that when he was comfortable, he was most powerful. It fueled my insides with daydreams of going back to California with him so that he could experience the soft grassy parks, moist air, and beautiful ocean sand.

Dip still had to be picked up frequently. And because he had an enlarged heart, we had to be extremely delicate with him. We couldn't just scoop him up by the tummy like a normal dog. It would put too much pressure on his chest and cause him to cough. I learned to raise his two little front paws and lean them onto the palms of my hands. Then I'd gently cup his butt with my other. It seemed to be working because his coughing lessened.

My little boy had his own personality and preferences by all means, and quickly caught on to how the treat thing worked. He saw how the other dogs begged for food, and who to cozy up to the most. Within days, Dip was cutting in line so that he could be the first to indulge. He'd even hang out where my stepdad sat because he realized that he was too weak to resist. He had those alluring eyes that made you melt and had you hand over your last bite at the same time.

He was picky though, and quite sure of himself. If he didn't like the food, he wouldn't eat it. If he didn't want to get up from bed, he didn't. If he wanted to eat what you were eating, he'd growl and bark until you gave it up. If he didn't like you, he'd let you know. He didn't have a single problem with showing you who he was. Self-expression was one of his finest characteristics. Yet, as strong and robust as parts of him appeared to be, he couldn't hide his gentle, fragile, loving nature when he slept. Never did I see him without a smile while in that dream dimension. He was another one of my angels and farthest from the "grumpy old man" that the idiot at the shelter tried to label him as. That experience just showed me that Dip wasn't getting treated right and he wasn't going to stand for it. So, good for him.

In just eight days, Dipper began running like a little puppy! He surprised us one afternoon by suddenly racing down the hallway. Then he added the living room, kitchen, and my bedroom to his escapades. He was a whole new dog with teen energy. We were speechless! We had no idea that a pet that age, and in those health conditions, could make that kind of transformation. Talk about a miracle! My stepdad was so captivated that he nicknamed him, "Vet."

Short for "Veteran," there were none of us who could relate more to the term than my stepdad. He served in Vietnam and had been surrounded by all levels, character, and ages of servicemen. Quickly on, he noticed symbolic similarities in Dipper, as we all did. Mostly, we couldn't get over the fact that he had survived 18 ½ years of life and was still going strong. He was showing us the importance of non-attachment, especially to labels that program us into thinking how our stories are supposed to finish out. Dip was completely the opposite. Nothing was going to stop him until he took his last breath, and that would only be here on this earth. You could tell that he'd go on and be just as illustrious in the spirit world. I had never met any being like him and I know my parents hadn't either. I had always said that ***"Age was nothing but a season. When you're given the opportunity to shine... you will surely blossom!"*** Thank goodness we were giving him back that opportunity. He was surely blossoming!

It had only been a month, and Dipper's frequency kept getting better. He was eating great, drinking tons of water, sleeping like a champion, and enjoying the outdoors. He exercised up and down the hallway, took walks on both sides of the property, licked my face like it was ice-cream, barked for food, and even growled at particular visitors. Like his sudden burst of energy that began three weeks earlier inside the trailer, he developed his second wave of zest outdoors. Every afternoon, when the clock struck 5:00 or 5:30pm, he'd run circles around everybody. He'd bolt from the bottom of the porch to the carport. Then he'd jet back to where the other set of stairs was. Sometimes he'd run after us. Other times, we'd run after him. When we'd catch him, we'd grab his butt and watch him dart out of our hands and into a new direction.

The other dogs also tried to join in. But I had to keep a close eye on Lola because I could tell she wanted to ambush him. He wasn't going to wait for anybody to figure things out though. He forgot about her venom and kept on sprinting until he had to stop for a minute to catch his breath. His smile from ear to ear was priceless. I didn't know if he was still jacked up on left-over meds from the shelter, or if he had that much natural dopamine flowing through his veins. Whatever it was, he was a rockstar and we wanted more of it!

I did notice that he had some issues with depth perception. On the day of his adoption, he almost walked off the passenger's seat and faceplanted onto the floormat. I didn't think anything of it because I knew he was loaded with meds and anesthesia. As time went on, I'd catch him walking in holes. He didn't care how to get from point A to point B; he just set his sights on point B. He'd run into branches and sometimes come back with a cactus, half the size of him, stuck in the front his neck. If I was building something outside and wood panels were scattered between us, he'd fall through every one of them just to get to where I was. He never took his eyes off the prize, literally. It was amazing how he'd be outside playing, sniffing the bushes, or exploring areas he shouldn't be anywhere near... and then I'd appear. His eyes would open wide, his ears would flap back, and he'd race right to me. No hole, bush, or cactus was going to get in his way.

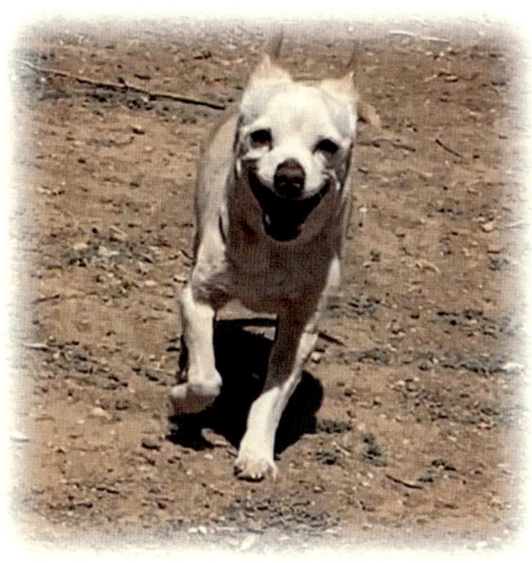

He knew I'd always be right by his side and was cognizant of that from the first time we met. Even though I left him in that facility for six days longer than I should have, he knew I was coming back. After bringing him home, he became aware that I wasn't going to let anything happen to him. I was his parent, caretaker, guide, protector, best friend, soulmate, and the pillar to help him become even better. Every day, he would show me the trust and love he had for me by leaning his ears into my hands whenever I massaged them.

We also had a shared trademark for affection. I would rub my nose into his fur like I was his animal mom who was sniffing out the previous day and caressing him with maternal nurturing. Sometimes I'd open my eyes to see if I could catch a glimpse of his expression. He would always have his lids closed while leaning into my face like a beautiful orange leaf in the middle of autumn... falling from the last tree of that season.

Sometimes he'd get lost in the moment. If I wasn't holding him up, his chin would gently fall to the floor. He'd stay frozen in the fairytale until the rest of his body crashed down. Oh, how he loved to have his little ears rubbed and chin nuzzled. Those were some of his prime acupressure points that I felt helped him produce happy hormones. As he came more into his own, his lungs strengthened. He began to roll on his back like a puppy so that I'd rub his tummy. He didn't have the strength to roll back over, so I had to take some precautions in making sure he never fell into a position where he could suffocate in his blankets. As time went on, that wouldn't be a worry. My little boy was evolving into a much stronger being, both mentally and physically. Maybe he embodied those superpowers all along and just had to be reminded like muscle memory. It was as if Dip was letting go and releasing past experiences and subconscious blocks that he may have never realized were anything important. He was opening himself up to the freedom of the present moment.

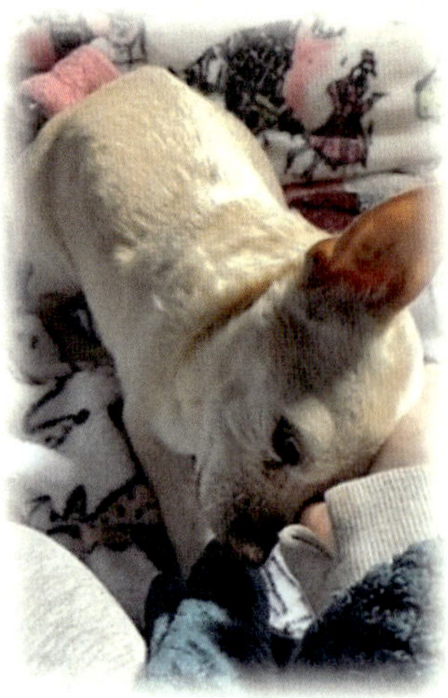
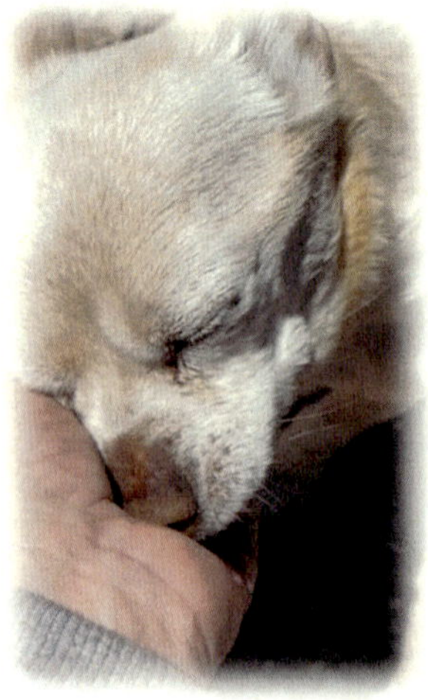

We had begun to develop a great routine together, not just with me, but for Bodhi, Lola, and Goldie. That meant my schedule completely modified into that of having a newborn. I had to get up with him many nights to pee and sometimes poop. All dogs had meal schedules, regimens, and formulas for tonics and health treatments. Food had to be prepped, water had to be replenished hourly, and Vaseline had to be rubbed on Dip's ears, nose, and penis. Butts would get baby-wiped, liquids got squirted into sides of gums, ointments had to be rubbed on Dip's tiny skin tags, eye boogers had to be cleaned, and beds had to be washed when peed in.

We were getting up between 5:30am and 6:30am, and knocked out by 9:30pm. Sometimes, he'd be out by 7pm sharp. Never in my life had I gone to sleep or woken up so early. Never had I realized all I could accomplish and experience that early in the morning. I was always the type of writer that did my best work in the late-night hours. "Vet" made me realize that, for so many years of my life, I had wasted valuable minutes sleeping. The more time I had with him, the better. Thank goodness I had begun taking pictures and videos of his every move. I had so many memories stored in my brain, but knew that I would want to go back and relive them someday.

Like all my dogs, Dip had to be right by me. If I was working on my laptop or doing some writing, he'd have to be within two feet of me. If he was in the bedroom napping, he'd choose the closest bed so that I'd be right there when he woke up. If I was trying to exercise on the porch, he'd stand right by the stationary bike or stretching mat. One of his bed cushions was based under an umbrella on the deck. So, sometimes he'd doze off while I took a break to tan. He slept deep and I was sure it had something to do with the comfy oasis I created for him on the floor. Sometimes he'd dream with his tongue out, sometimes he'd sprawl his biology over two beds, sometimes he'd pick a spot on the floor, and sometimes he'd snore. But always, he'd smile. He didn't spend the nights on my bed, but we invested plenty of other times there laying close together. He'd snuggle up to my face, stare into my eyes, and tell me over and again how thankful he was. Before I'd get to thank him back, he'd pass out on my arm. An hour later, I'd be numb.

I had to believe that the experience was a rebirth for Dip. Dogs his age and health status weren't usually given second chances. As a developing natural healer over the previous 20-sum years, I had learned how mind, thought, belief, and perception could influence the physical aspects of our well-being. Dip was evolving into something I couldn't have dreamt of. I had never doubted those powers in humans. I just had no idea that an animal could be as phenomenal. He was indeed beating the odds and leading us all by example.

One of the miracles I was extremely proud of was the progressive development with his vertebrae. In less than a week, his protruding hump had gone down immensely. His abdomen began deflating and his legs strengthened so much that his backbone started to straighten. My stepdad couldn't believe it. I remembered the look on his face the day I brought Dip home. I knew he thought I made a big mistake because of how sick he looked. But within days, he was taking on a new shape. It was like his structure was correcting itself. I posted pictures to show the incredible impact that adoption can make on an animal's life and the powerful manifestations of love and nurture. People were in awe. The first photo on the top left was taken on the fourth day Dipper was with us. The last photo on the bottom right was captured less than twelve weeks later. I wrote this message next to one of his before-and-after posts: "If a spine can shift in three months, can you imagine would else can?!"

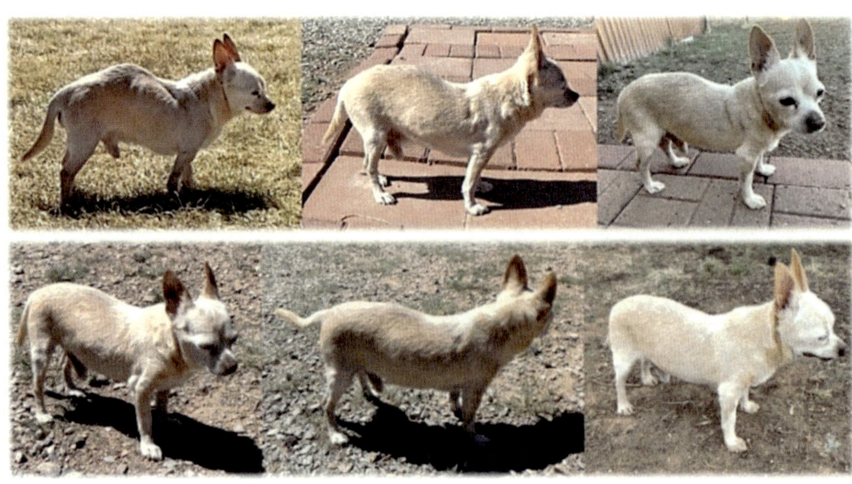

Not many dogs make it to 18 ½ years of age, much less their eyesight and cognizance. My dog had both. He knew to stay close, knew where his safe space was, and still had his motor skills. When he'd wander off a little too far from where I was working, all I had to do was call out his name and take a few steps in his direction. He'd turn around, see me instantly, and sprint right to me. Although sometimes, he'd actually run right by me. LOL!

As much as I thought I needed him to hear my voice, I began seeing it as a blessing that he couldn't. He felt it instead. He undoubtedly recognized my call for him. And when I'd give him commands, most of the time, he'd respond. I knew that he had some type of auditory stimulus, whether it be purely tone, sound, or vibration. My mom would be outside playing with him and, the minute I'd walk out the front door, he would try to find where the pitch of my voice was coming from. If I didn't say a word, he'd still feel the vibes of my footsteps no matter if I was on top of the deck and he was underneath. He would find me every single time. There were other instances where he'd be in a sleep coma in my room, and the second I'd open the fridge, he'd peek around the corner to see what I was cooking. His sensory perceptions were so intact that he could smell, hear, and feel the thought of food.

I had to admit, there were plenty of other instances when Dip didn't hear a thing. I could clap and scream my loudest, and he wouldn't flinch. I actually loved that quality because it allowed him to go at his own speed without having to hear all the bullshit in the world. Fireworks didn't faze him and gun shots didn't scare him. He'd simply chill or sleep through it all. Just like humans, he probably had selective hearing. He was likely laughing at us the entire time and thinking, *"Why do they keep talking to me like I'm a baby?"*

As he got stronger and his lungs got healthier, he started playing in his covers. I stepped away for a few minutes to put some clothes in the washer one time. When I came back, he was nowhere. I checked the whole house and still no Dip. I was sick to my stomach. After spotting movement, I found him dug under three layers of blankets in his corner floor cushion. It was amazing to see him being so playful, but it probably caused me to have an underlying ulcer.

When it came to leaving the house for anything, Dipper almost always went with me. He needed to be tended to hourly, so I couldn't leave him home alone for longer than a morning. Bodhi used to fill that spot and I missed that. But he was gaining some independence of his own since Lola had come into the picture. I could run errands in town and not have to worry about him crying for hours. He was my shadow, don't get me wrong. But he and Lola were becoming buddies and finding their own formulas. I knew Bodhi missed our formulas, but I also reassured him constantly that we would get back to ourselves again one day. I knew that he understood.

Since Dip was so easy going, it was just as easy traveling with him. I bought a shoulder sling so that he'd be comfy strolling through the stores with me. If I had a meeting, I'd bring his bed and he'd snuggle into it and relax for the entire time we were there. There was one instance when I was getting acupuncture and he just couldn't stand to see needles embedded in my skin. He fussed until my practitioner picked him up and placed him next to my face where he could make sure I wasn't getting hurt. Dip went to auditions with me and actually joined me in my introductory slates. He also starred in the second to last audition I went on locally. If anybody had the "X" factor, it was him. If I was ever going to book an acting job, it was going to be because of him. He made me look that good and believe that I was that good. We made the perfect team and were accomplishing our to-do lists together. Where dogs weren't allowed to go, we didn't go.

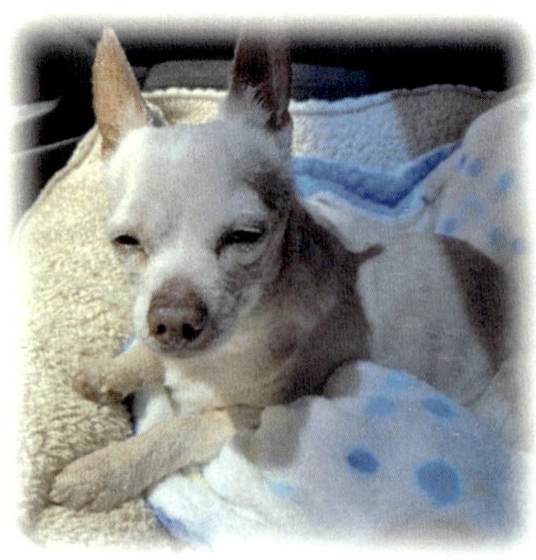

Sometimes, he'd stay up for the drive home, sometimes he'd sleep all the way back, and most of the time, he wanted to sit on my lap. He enjoyed the comfort of his bed in the passenger seat, but nothing soothed his Root and Heart chakras more than being right next to me. He'd cuddle in between the steering wheel for part of the drive, then sit up on my knee so that he could look out and enjoy the scenery. As we'd cross the underpass, Dip would get a rush of excitement. I'd roll down the window, pick him up, and let him stick his head out. For the next mile, he'd breathe in that fresh mountain air.

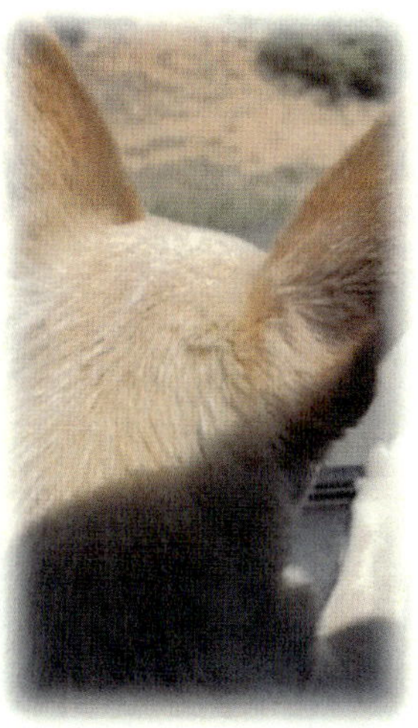

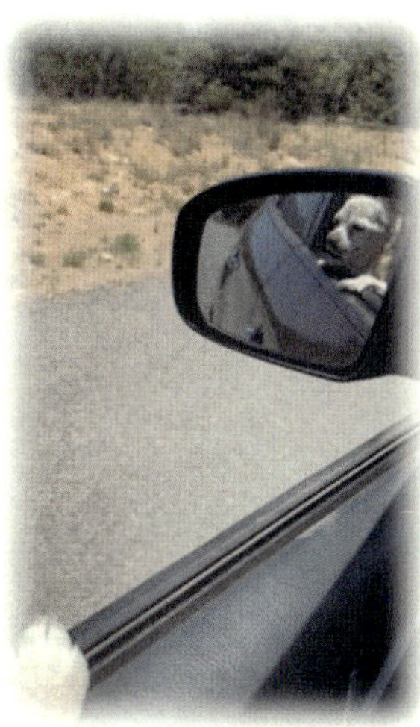

The few times Dip didn't cruise with me, I was fortunate enough to have my stepdad watch him for the hours I was gone. On the weekends that I'd have to go into town to buy them food and supplements, it would be my mom. Those two were hysterical and were the epitome of grandparents. Sometimes I'd come home to see the gate up in my room and Dip stumped face down in one of his beds as if he was in solitary confinement. Other times, he'd be sleeping in a cushion all by himself in the middle of the living room with chaos all around him. I'd catch my mom feeding him hard dog food and pieces of steak the size of his front leg. They'd give him processed treats that I specifically advised against and had him outside with Goldie running dust circles around him. I'd be pissed, but then appreciative that he was still alive by the time I made it home.

As good as his good days were, Dip also had down times. His cough would come and visit, he'd lose energy, get diarrhea, and sometimes gag up clear liquid. There were days his tummy was swollen, his back was arched, and he'd nap for hours. A few times, he painfully panted after eating, and a few others, he wouldn't eat at all. A few instances, he lost his balance and walked in a semi-circle with his head tilted. Some nights, we'd just sit in his bed on the floor together for hours, or take walks through the hallway at 4am. Other nights, we'd go outside and stand in the cool breeze, even if the rain showed up. He loved the smell of the drizzle and how the fresh droplets soaked his fur. Every one of those nights, we'd see the Little Dipper shining down on us. It was ethereal how those stars would connect with my little boy. He was just as cosmic as Bodhi, but in his own special way.

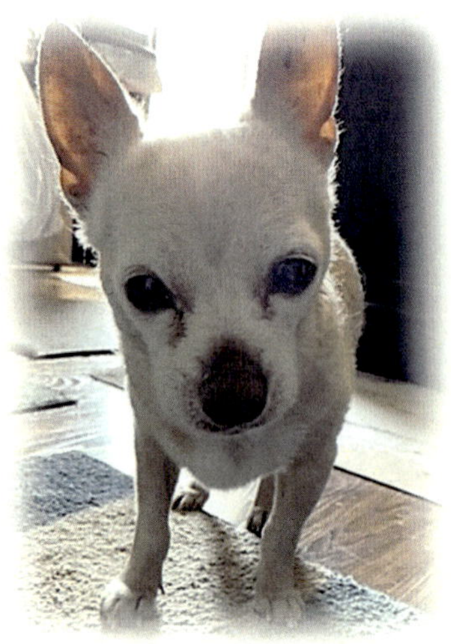

As tough as those days were, he'd always bounce back almost immediately. There were only four times when his ailments required more than my research and natural treatments. Three were common conditions. Whereas, the fourth required a lump to be removed from the back of his right thigh that the vet had missed on his first visit. She was able to cut out the nodule without putting him under anesthesia. It was so comfy that he fell asleep while she performed the surgery. I will forever be grateful for the gentle approach she took in making that happen. She added a potential eighteen months to his life!

It was interesting how much I was learning about him, our connection, and myself through our anatomies, and how they responded to everything. I never realized how a human could be so much like a dog since dogs were so much better than us. We were light years away from developing aspects remotely close to them. In no way could I have ever ultimately reached Dip's level of soulness, but we both had double chins and probably the same amount of white hair growing underneath them. Neither of us did well with too many supplements no matter how healthy or organic. We both did better with nutritional food and the natural process of digestion.

When it came to prescription medication, it was lethal for the both of us. Although the veterinarian that removed his lump was always extremely kind and gentle with him, she'd get out of hand with the pharmaceuticals. On two of our visits, she sent him home with potent drugs, including a narcotic. Every time, he'd slump over, lose mobility, and deteriorate. Those drugs didn't help him; they removed life from him. He was a dog who just didn't do well with them in any dosages. My body experienced almost the exact reactions in my past as well. I knew myself, and had the power of autonomy. But Dip was a 100% dependent on me. I always knew better not to take that route with him. Yet, I wasn't a veterinarian. The ultimate goal was always to help him, even if that meant trying something different.

Another intriguing factor of our connection was with our backbones and digestive systems. Dipper had kyphosis possibly from age, toxicity, pancreatitis, tumors, viruses, gastrointestinal disease, or injury. I had vertebral compression fractures and deformities to T7 and T8 from my 1989 automobile accident, which led to mild scoliosis through the lower thoracic part of my spine. Some of his other sporadic symptoms indicated that his pancreas might've also played a role in other areas than just his dorsal curvature. I, too, had developed a sensitive dual organ from the same collision, which continually plagued my assimilation of food and emotional nutrients over the years. It was either due to the blow that I took from being compressed out of the window as I was ejected, or it was one of the areas I'd been storing my hidden worry and trauma in. Nevertheless, we both had similar systems that were imbalanced and problematic.

I never had to get up at night to use the restroom until I entered my past relationship. It was as if my kidneys were detoxing my system from all of the daily stress, and drawing out the emotional phlegm that built up in my air pumps. I had returned to a healthy kidney yin, bladder balance, and got some breath back by the time Bodhi came into my life. But when Dipper arrived, I began frequently urinating again. I didn't understand it at the time, but signs would come to me later that I was likely flushing the fluid out of his lungs for him.

How cool was it to be connected on levels where our bodies could help each other? The stars did it all the time. Him and I were linked just as intergalactically, but in different forms. It made me love our alone times that much more, especially when we'd walk outside and sit on the front steps soaking in the soft sun rays and cool breeze. The birds would be chirping and the sky would whistle sweet nothings. It had been a place of solace for me before him, and now it was more meaningful with him.

I saw how relaxed and trusting he was with me in those moments. His calmness was exquisite. Seeing him enjoy the eccentricities of nature brought us that much closer. She was our Mother, both in form and in spirit, bonded together. As we sat with her, she'd reminisce on how beautiful the process of everything truly was, no matter the illusions. She'd give us signs, forms of light, and footprints of where we were headed next. With every totem she sent, Dip and I would sit in serenity and embrace the quality of every message.

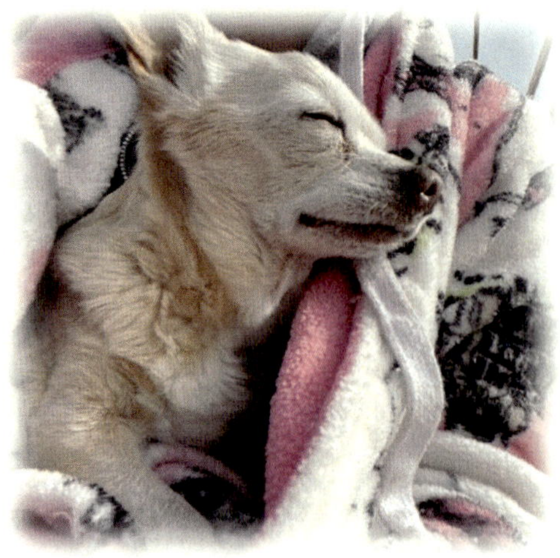

I had to give credit to my lil Bodhi, because he was forced to take a back seat to Dipper. He was my original road dog, my one and only, and the sweet pea who I did everything with. I felt so bad every time I looked into his eyes and saw how much he missed me. I'd kiss his adorable little face and tell him how much I loved him and appreciated all he was doing. His eyes would sparkle back with a look of understanding that he knew Dipper required so much more than him. That was Bodhi, and that was why he was so special to all of us.

He knew the formula had changed, but also knew that we were doing a great thing for Dip; for the collective. Lola had been keeping him busy anyway. Her moods reflected a Mercury Retrograde cycle and he was trying to figure her out. Within a month of having her, we got her spayed in hopes of taming her rage. She was a terrorizer and had attacked Dipper one more time inside the house, and another on the day of her surgery. I was so irate that I thought about rehoming her. I had been completely disconnected and didn't even like her.

I couldn't really fault her because we adopted her three days before Dipper. She never really got the chance to bond with me and quickly became the middle child who nobody paid attention to. Dip was the new little baby who had all eyes on him. Bodhi got demoted to second in line. That meant even less intervals for her. I was glad that I saved her life, but I thought I had jumped in too quickly. Luckily, my mom had an extra soft spot for her. I knew that when I'd go back to LA, I'd be okay with leaving her. She had become a country dog and didn't want anything to do with being inside. She barked at everything, rolled around in the weeds, chased the sound of neighboring cars, and enjoyed every ounce of freedom that my parents' property offered her. She wouldn't have lasted in an apartment.

She ended up settling down a bit and began showing similar traits of the other dogs. She learned a few nicknames like, "Lolies" – "Loes" – "Loles" – and "Lolita." She also started rolling on her back to get her belly rubbed. No matter if she was on gravel, dirt, shit, or weeds, that became her trademark for affection. We knew that she was different from the very beginning, so her unique styles of love were no surprise. She was still ferocious, and displayed her two racks of sharp fangs on a daily basis. But she actually began looking like a cute dog.

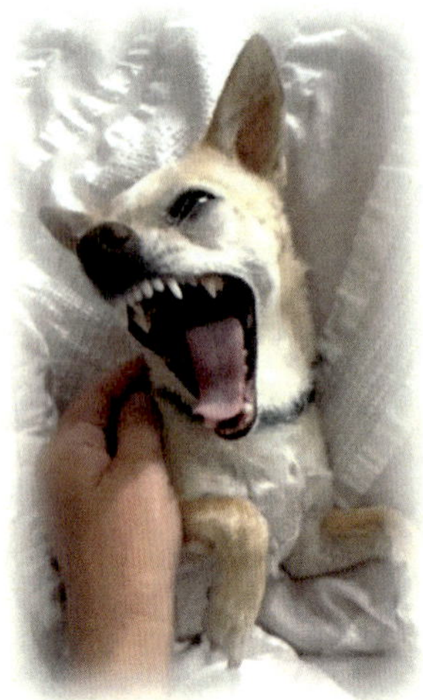 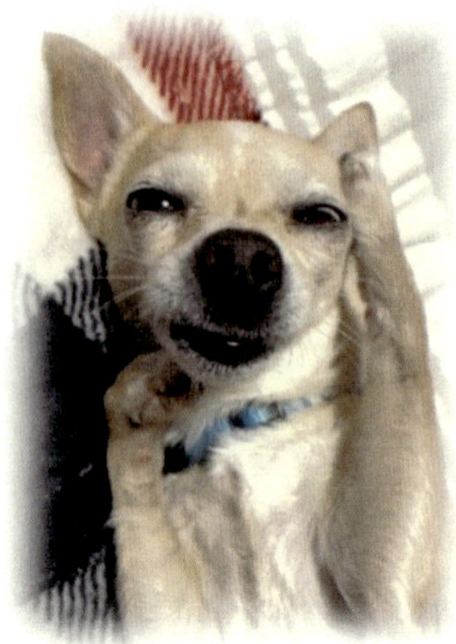

She also hung out on the bathroom rug while I showered, and would lick the water off my legs afterwards just like Charly used to do. Whereas Bodhi became a serial tail wagger, Lola turned into a serial licker. You'd have to keep her away from the expensive vitamin E oil on your face. She'd also manage to sit on the back end of the couch to give my stepdad a personal head and ear wash in ten-minute increments. She ate when she wanted and that was usually when she could rub it in Goldie's face. Other times, she'd haul her food into the living room to eat with everyone else. Then she wouldn't have an ounce of shame engaging in romantic relations with her doggy cushion while we sat there watching.

She was on her own time and mood schedule, and absolutely didn't need to be coddled. She'd curl up on the pillow at the corner of the sofa and moan when you'd ask her if something was wrong. Then annoying Goldie would strut by and instigate a fight by carrying a toy she'd been playing with earlier. That's when the princess would turn diabolical. I didn't think it was anything personal. She was just a territorial dog in general. Her previous homelife probably included having to fight for food. I wished she didn't have to go through that, but I seemed to be the only one bothered by it. Just when I'd begin to feel sorry for her, she'd move on to something else. By the next morning, she'd be outside with Goldie causing a ruckus all over again.

Out of all the dogs, Lola was the only one who did what she was told. She undeniably knew her name and never went against my commands. She also loved playing with any toy you could throw for her to fetch back. You would've never known that she was 12 years old. I knew there was a spark of playfulness and spunk underneath that protective exterior. She just had to go at her own pace to get acclimated. I began to learn that she also had a custom way of settling into her safe space. Like us humans, there was no timeline for her healing or recovery. Who knew all that she went through before coming into our lives? All we could do was continue providing her with safety, trust, and comfort. It would be up to her when she would harmonize with the rest of the group.

It didn't help that Goldie would irritate her to the max. I started to think it was a girl thing because the jealousy was evident. But it seemed like it actually gave Lola a sense of purpose and empowerment. Goldie was unattached. She wouldn't let some pointy incisors ruin any part of her day. She'd utilize the windows of pestering when she could, but then she'd go with the flow and continue doing her own thing. Yet, Lola still made it a point to put up blocks for her. And in the process, Goldie's indirect influence began allowing her to shift moods. She was still a full-fledged Wicked Witch of the East one minute, but would transform into a cute cuddle bunny the next. This was coming from a doggy who was abused by an owner that she only knew as someone who adored her all the other years of having her.

Lola wasn't the only one benefiting from Goldie's nauseating energy with a newfound liveliness. Bodhi was also budding. I started to see a new level of confidence emerging within him. His stance was more upright, he began holding his ground when Goldie tried to steal his toys, he'd walk over to visit my stepdad by himself, and he'd bark in the nighttime darkness as if protecting us from something on the other side of the gate. It was exciting to see him gain some form of individuality. The self-assurance was beginning to beam through every pore in his system, and the golden hue in his satin fur was symbolic of the strength and balance he had built up inside of his Solar Plexus. He even developed his own upbeat strut. My little Bodes was growing into an incredible young dog, and I was so proud of him.

I even caught him trying to hump Goldie a few times. I was pleased that he wanted to use the balls he thought he had left, but I felt that he could do better. She was too big and boisterous for him. Plus, she broke wind on a regular basis and tossed her cookies just as often. His and Lola's friendship was platonic, so that wasn't in the cards either. Yet, I felt that he'd match up with a dog a bit closer to his size, age, and mellow mannerisms. She could be an eccentric hippy who was just as easy going, free-spirited, and had a healthier digestive system. He definitely wouldn't do well with anyone controlling.

He was a stud muffin and steadily grounding into the roots of his meaning and mission. I could see how good it made him feel that he was able to do things on his own. He was always going to whine for food and practically throw up in his muzzle from barely cutting the tips of his nails. He was also still going to need me to hold his paws in the snow when winter came back to visit. He'd for sure never stop crying like a baby every time I'd return home; knowing that I didn't abandon him. And although he had bad dreams often, I knew they'd eventually fade away as he got more settled in. Charly and Tippet used to have nightmares as well. I always wondered what was in their little minds, and if they were affected by the toxicity in that household. When it came to Bodes, I just prayed he wasn't haunted from his recent experience with his previous human. Luckily, I'd gently shake him enough to wake him up, so that he could come back to himself. No matter the trances, he no longer needed me to be with him on every step of our walks. He didn't need me to go with him to pee, and I could leave him home knowing that he was at peace.

The plan was working out just like I intended. Of all the dogs, I had to thank Lola. Not only was she playing a pivotal role in helping Bodhi, but she was helping Dipper. Because of her, I was able to give him all of my attention. And because of that, he had evolved into an incredibly healthy being. I no longer pulsated with anger over his shelter experience and wasn't as upset at the owner who gave him up. I was enthralled with continuing to extend the quality of his story. I loved watching him enjoy life and how he'd send me signs and messages about my own. One of his most constructive kept showing up and I couldn't deny that it was something I finally had to face.

8
The Soular System: Aligning With True Bliss

I had been so smitten with the fulfillment of Dipper that I began thinking less about being on camera and anything to do with Los Angeles. That space was becoming distant. I didn't miss the entitlement, greed, social pressure, sexual harassment, and politics of that business and parts of that city. Nor, did I miss the lack of auditions and being overlooked for how I didn't look. I was tired of the cattiness, shadiness, constant rejection, ongoing grind, and the lack of a guaranteed paycheck. I was also no longer submerged in the disconnectedness and wondering daily if I was ever going to make it. Plus, it was nice to be away from all the insecurity and a culture of not being able to age gracefully.

I did, however, long for the food, weather, ocean, palm trees, golf courses, beautiful homes, and the diversity. You could be a yuppie rockstar, tattoo artist, poet, athlete, teacher, or plumber, and you'd find groups that were just as similar. I missed the endless possibilities of startups and the degree of professionalism. My hometown was known as "The Land of Manana" because people operated when they could, not when they should. Plus, many times, corners would get cut. There was no half-assing of anything in that sunshine city.

Although the cultivation of money could be obnoxious, I craved the collective abundant mentality. They didn't think poor out there, and not just monetarily. That place was filled with a fresh glow, expert health treatments, spiritual healers, and pet lovers. The parks were gorgeous and I'd tan and earth at my favorite on Roxbury Drive. I also loved the amazing comedy clubs. There surely wasn't anything boring about Tinseltown and the excitement was infectious. Yet, it was nice having the option to go out if I wanted, or chill at home if I didn't. I yearned for those good aspects of my life, but even more for the few close connections I made. They were gems and I missed them dearly.

I hadn't spoken to many of my friends back in LA in quite some time, much less anyone those days. Not only was I secluded from society, but the topography was costing me my physical appearance. The closest gym was over twenty miles away, and beauty salons and organic grocers were forty. The massive number of Juniper trees and pollen caused me to develop some serious allergies. My face had been swollen for almost two months. My eyes were bloodshot. And a recurring irritation developed on the inside of my nose from blowing so much. I was just begging the Universe to bless us with consistent rain so that I could literally breathe again.

It was weird because I felt like one side of me was perfectly happy, but the other side wasn't. I had Dipper, yet I couldn't stand where I lived. I was free of any pressure to work, yet I longed for the hype of success that creativity fueled me with. I detested the way I felt and looked, yet Dip kept showing me that my value to the world came through so many other gifts than just my outside surface. I had so much more to offer, and in so many other ways. So, why did a part of me feel miserable, and why was I still hanging on to my profession?

Maybe it was because LA was all I knew and the stage for some of my biggest thrills. It was all I had done, lived, inhaled, and believed in as an adult. Or maybe, it was because I never felt aligned with where I grew up. Other than being a scholastic student and star athlete as a kid, and winning a few bikini contests in college, nothing fueled my inner being in New Mexico except for my parents. I cherished the years I got to live and evolve with them. Hence, I couldn't ever discount all of my time in that dry-climate state as being a downer.

I knew that I was upset for coming back almost four years earlier. Even though LA wasn't working for me, I was angry that I completely took myself out of my element and allowed my whole life to be changed. More so, I was disappointed in where I ended up because of it. The regret that wedged itself in my diaphragm felt like a bowling ball. I had no idea what else I could do, should do, or would have to do in order to eat and pay bills. Maybe I was scared to take a different direction and have to do something that I couldn't identify with. I didn't have anywhere else to go but to a place I thought I knew... and so badly wanted to leave a place I felt forcibly planted in.

I had to ask myself if it was it worth diving back into that pool? I had just turned 47 years of age. I wasn't improving my personal economy where I was currently living, but could I even make it in LA anymore? Did I even want to? How could I go back into an industry that marketed to a much younger generation, and with my so-so resume? The last thing I wanted to do was struggle. I had no desire to chase a dream, or beg others to buy me and my products. I certainly wasn't going to be a slave to any business again.

I also had to factor in that I had three new fur kids, including one who required 24-hour care. My goals had changed and, therefore, I'd have to consider only the jobs that would be compatible with having them. When it really came down to it, I wasn't thinking about moving because of a job. I couldn't imagine doing anything else or being anywhere else than with Dipper. The only thing I had was my present moment. That was his most prominent feature. It just didn't come easy, because I couldn't get over thinking that I needed to move him to a better place. I had to seriously take into account whether I really missed LA, and believed it would be more beneficial for him... or if I just wanted to get out of New Mexico. It wasn't about me anymore.

By mid-June, I was two months into a lawsuit against my ex for allegedly swindling me out of acquisitions we made as a couple. When I had confronted him in October of the previous year, I couldn't mentally handle his responses. It was eight months later and Dip was the difference maker. His extraordinary transformation had inspired me so much that I gained back the strength to stand up for myself.

I had also helped to complete a remarkable remodel of my stepdad's bathroom as well as a posh porch deck and cover for my mom. I was surprisingly advancing in other areas besides entertainment. I wrote when I could, still kept up on the landscaping and technical issues of both households, and continued to post on *Furever Soulmates*. Yet, my emphasis was always on Dipper. He had evolved into something spectacular. His soft fur had almost fully grown back on both sides of his ears. He had no more crusties or discoloration on his dermis layer. And most pigmentation and age spots had faded. If he could fly, his auricles would've been his wings. They were a clear indication of how optimal his health had become.

His spine had straightened even more, and his raw, tender, red skin under his chin had thickened. He was nowhere close to resembling anything pink. Instead, he was a dazzling cream-colored white glow as that of an Arabian Horse. He had no apparent issues with his abdomen; that too had flattened. He didn't whine in pain, wheeze when sleeping, or have any troubles breathing. He even stopped peeing in the bed at night, and could hold his bladder for more than eight hours at a time. When I picked him up, there was no more cracking of his bones. It was as if his skeleton had morphed into a steel frame. His back legs extended, his posture heightened, and his youthful vibrance amplified through his surface. He was maintaining balance. He had great days and still a few not-so-great ones. Sometimes he looked and acted older. And most other times, he looked and acted like a puppy. Nobody would've ever believed he was the same dog three months earlier.

There was something in the stars for him. I remember coming back from his acupuncture session one afternoon and seeing my odometer at 77777. He was sitting right by me in the passenger seat as calm as could be. The day was June 16th. It was another reminder of that lucky energy that kept following his path. I knew that 2021 was going to continue being the best year of our lives and, inevitably, good fortune and health would continue to bless us all for many more to come!

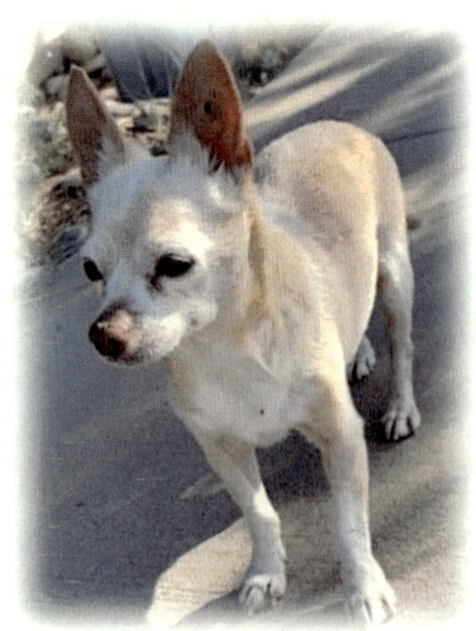

We had reached fly, mosquito, and ant season, and they sure did rule the world. Those disturbing critters could penetrate through anything, even the barriers of skin and fur. My mom never got bitten because she drank a tablespoon of apple cider vinegar with lemon and warm water every morning. Those bugs hated that sour taste and stayed far away, but came after me instead. No matter how much peppermint, lemongrass, and eucalyptus essential oils I'd spray all over the room and my body, I'd wake up in the morning with throbbing boulders on my forehead and neck from getting munched on throughout the night. I couldn't even lay out in the sun for more than ten minutes to tan without them coming out to attack the coconut oil lathered all over my skin. The evening hours were their main feeding times. Yet, those were prime hours for Dip to be able to stay outside longer because it was cooler. As much as they bothered me, I wasn't going to allow them to shift Dip's schedule. That meant doing whatever it took to divert them.

I would leave the front screen door open so that he could walk in and out as he pleased. I'd sit on the step while he'd stand snuggled next to my leg, watching the morning sunrise turn into noon time. Then he'd walk right to the edge of one of the porch's two staircases and ooze in contentedness. Most of our 24-hours were spent down on the bottom step of the front staircase enjoying all we could of the sunlight. He'd graze in the yard, eat some dirt, and then chill underneath the trailer deck with Bodhi, Lola, and Goldie. Always, he'd end up peaking his darling little face through the steps so that he could be a part of the experience. He loved it outside.

As summer was about to set in, it meant hotter temps. I noticed he began to pant occasionally. So, no matter how much he wanted to stay outdoors, I had to take preventative measures. I consistently kept him cool, sprinkled moist water on the top of his head, and made sure he had plenty of drinking water. I wanted to do all I could to keep anything from hindering his delicate heart, as well as avoiding stroke and exhaustion. Yet, no matter the geology, we made the fresh air a priority. That front door stayed open so that he could enjoy as much self-sufficiency as possible. All it meant was having more itchy bites, and shorter lifespans for the insect trespassers.

The more freedom I gave Dip, the better. He'd go out to the porch on his own, but always made sure to stay nearby. He would peek his head in and just stand there looking at me, while I was writing on my laptop at the corner of the bar top. He was making sure I wasn't going anywhere. He couldn't walk down the steps or climb up, but on a few occasions, he'd get down them. I remember one time taking my eyes off of him for only a few minutes. Then I spotted him across the yard taking a dump next to the front gate. He either made it to the bottom level slowly and safely, or he rolled down at the cost of his organs, spine, and bones. He actually fell through the steps one time right in front of me. I hadn't pulled the blinds down far enough, and he was trying to crawl under so that he could get closer to the sun. I was a second too late in grabbing him. I remember seeing how much he ached afterward, but he didn't want to admit it. I couldn't live with myself if I ever contributed to hurting him in any way.

By July, he was thriving at miraculous levels and, shockingly, becoming independent. I could leave him out front while he sniffed the several patches of grass that suddenly popped up. He'd also mark his spots and soak in the sun for a bit. His back limbs had become so strong that, on occasion, he'd lift his leg to pee on the weeds and cement blocks. Sometimes, he'd even mark Goldie. It was epic!!! I had seen the same progress with Bodhi who was almost sixteen years younger. Witnessing Dipper made it all such a combined better.

In so many ways, he was becoming my mentor. Not just to me, but to all of us. Being in the present moment was the most essential of his lessons and the most authentic of his characteristics. He wouldn't be anywhere else on the planet, but with you. He also showed us the importance of letting shit go and forgetting, as life was too short and too small not to get along. He demonstrated that with Lola. Her aggressive behavior towards him in the beginning never fazed him. He'd still be friends with her the next day and, many times, leading the way. His energy was contagious. She even softened up and desperately wanted him to reciprocate the same friskiness.

But as playful as Dipper could be, he'd never get out of his lane. He stuck to what made him happiest. That was the type of honesty and substance he represented within. Nothing was superficial about him.

He'd been there, and done that, so he didn't need to be in a hurry to do anything else. Life wasn't a race and none of us knew how long we had left anyway. There was no point in missing out what was in front of us, while being too busy looking ahead to a future not guaranteed.

There was no doubt that Dip was bluntly expressive. That was probably why he gravitated to his blue blanket, which represented his 5th Throat chakra. He was about communication, speech, and self-purity. It actually brought me back to my beautiful Blue. I knew there was a keen connection between the two of them. It wasn't just the color, but how poetic they were in showing their truths. Maybe a part of Blue's ethereal spirit quantumly jumped into part of Dip's. There were many times I could magically see his image in Dipper's shadows while taking walks at my mom's office. I knew Blue would always be with us in some form of my dogs. The name and color of his psyche just happened to interlace into Dip's thyroid. It was obvious that the connection originated below in the 4th Heart chakra, since it interlinked Dip's hormones, emotions, love, and balance. He was a warmhearted being who loved unconditionally. His core was open and brilliant like the emerald crystal of my birthday gemstone. That's probably why he was also drawn to his green blankie.

In the first few months, I had picked up some Blue Calcite and Mookaite crystals. I placed them in Dip's beds to help sooth his immune system with comfort, strength, and relaxation. I felt that the baby blue rocks could help calm emotions and offer mental protection. One of the crystals was a large heart-shaped type of love nucleus in which I placed in his main bed next to where I slept. The burgundy stones were to help ground his mind, heart, and soul, and continue helping him to live in the moment. Something was working, because he had no problem in any of those areas.

My original intent was to get Dipper out of the shelter so he wouldn't die there. I didn't think he had much time left, so I wanted his last days, or weeks, or months, or even years, to be the best he ever had. Yet, there was so much more to that adoption than just predicting and soothing his ending. He was bringing me back to the center of my own being. He was helping to peel off the layers of illusions and attachments from my past learned perceptions.

Dipper was my mirror and the epitome of purpose and meaning. Everything about him, his space, and his energy, mattered. His spiritual messages, magnetic personality, resilience, fragileness, and his originality were captivating. He taught me so many things in the simplest form; so many lessons that I thought I had already fine-tuned. Being in his presence was Godlike, and trust that I had never fully coordinated my beliefs with a central form of a higher source. I had been challenged numerous times throughout my life whether there was that type of existence at all.

My creator and guide had always been Mother Nature. After coming into contact with Dip, I knew that he was that force. He rooted life back into me and provided the flooring for my foundation and security. Like the photosynthesis of a plant, he was the light that fueled me with nutritional elements. I knew that Dip knew how vital he had been to my survival. We shared that kind of connective bond where neither one of us had to say a word, or bark. We both just knew and felt the emotions behind every touch and expression. Every single day I would sit down with him face-to-face. As I looked into his beautiful brown lenses, he would tell me that I was the best thing that had ever happened to him. I would always smile back... and tell him that I felt the same way about him.

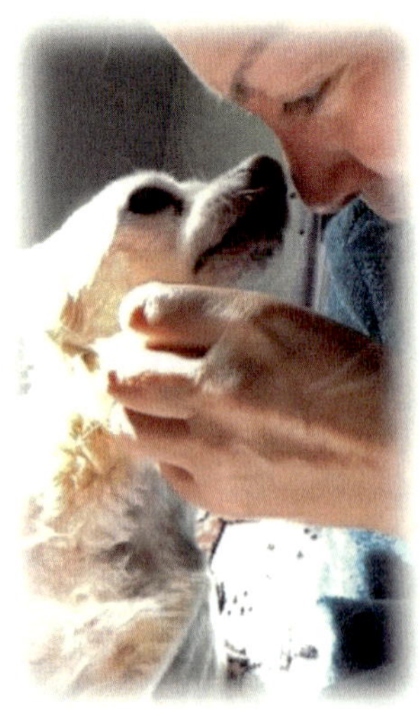

Dipper was always drawn to the light. Some days he'd walk into the office, or into my mom's bedroom, and just stand there looking towards the windows. At certain hours during the afternoon, he'd walk down the hallway when beams of brilliance would shine down the corridor like a stained-glass chapel. It was no different when he'd be outside soaking in the rays. I didn't know if he was corresponding with some form of artificial intelligence, ghosts, angels, or even spirits. Or, if simply, a higher light and higher source were calling him.

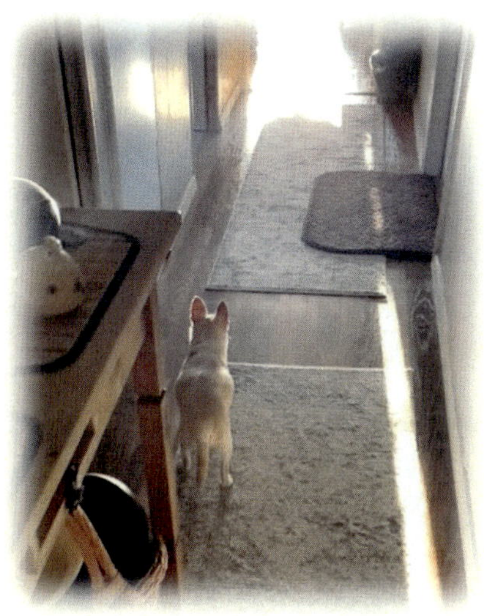

Sometimes I wondered what he was thinking as I'd watch him lay in his bed, with his eyes open, looking into space. I wondered if he thought about why his family abandoned him and stuck him in a cage to die alone. Or, why parts of his body were letting him down. Or, why a shelter neutered him when they didn't have to. And because so, he was going to suffer painful coughs and lifelong problems. I wondered if he thought about how he got where he did in life, and how he was relocated into an even better place with us. I wondered if he believed in karma and how confusing it was to understand when he didn't do anything to deserve it. Or maybe, he felt the blessings that he was receiving from the positive side of it. I wondered if he knew how much time he had left and how I would handle it. I wondered, if he wondered, how much I'd miss him when it happened. No, I knew he knew that answer. I just wondered if he knew something I didn't.

I wondered on those days, when he didn't feel so well, if those would be our last moments together. I would cry and cry. I had grown so much with him, evolved with him, gained contentedness and acceptance with him, and loved him so abundantly... that I couldn't lose him. I couldn't imagine life without him. Yet, I forgot that dogs died too. I forgot that I brought him home with us so that he could go peacefully someday. I just never wanted to think of that someday. I got caught up in the notion that I could have him forever. That thought pattern allowed me to live to the absolute fullest with him. Every single moment I had with Dip, I lived like it was his last.

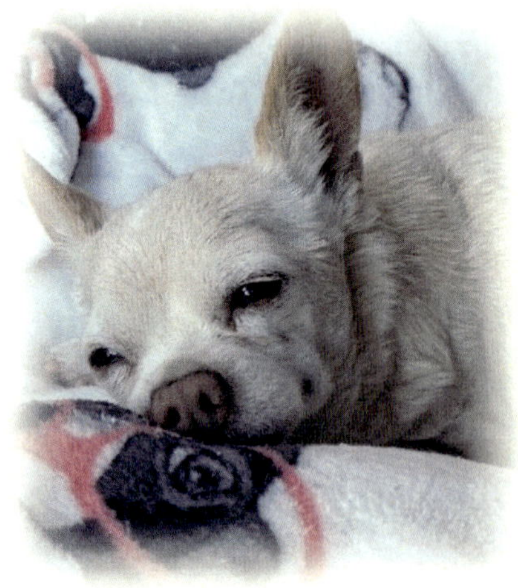

The mindset carried over to the rest of the dogs because they were also thriving to the fullest. Even the cat and canines on the other side of the property had brought magnificence to the table. Everybody played a role. Bodhi's had unfortunately minimized and it was a tough pill to swallow. I felt Dip's recovery to be more of a life and death situation than his 3-year-young vibrant self. I knew there were no guarantees for the period of time we'd ever have with our pets. But in the core of that moment, I felt it was more probable that I'd have Bodhi longer than Dipper, and progressively healthier. I was unwaveringly sure that I was making the right choices for the best of everyone, not just Dip. It may have come at the price of my attention. But, in the long run, I knew we'd all benefit.

I made sure to make a conscious effort daily to keep Bodhi from ever feeling any less important. No matter how absent I was in the way I was, I always made it known that he was my number one. Although I was giving all my time to Dip, he was my closest. He got seniority on all treats. He got to sit right next to me on the couch when we would have our meals. He got the best compliments and tummy massages, and he had the ultimate sleeping position on my bed. That was his spot, and always his spot, no matter where the Universe took any of us. He was my soul child, and every single night we'd continue to snuggle face-to-face while doing our prayers and meditation on our way into sleep mode.

Some nights, I'd catch myself falling back into the same old "being stuck" mind sores. Bodhi was always there to listen. I'd complain about how everyone in my household, and in that entire desert state, spoke so poorly of LA. I'd vent about the residual checks of twenty years' worth of work going from thousands of dollars to cents. I'd always bring up how the dust, wind, weeds, foxtails, and the climate of the demographic were becoming a huge problem. My entire aura was so dried out that my mind, spirit, and bones were cracking. My skin went from supple to parched. Deep wrinkles and lines formed, spider veins emerged, my knees decayed, and the heels of my feet molded into the pretenses of calluses. Most of me felt crepey like dried superglue, whereas other parts kept crumbling like rocks falling down mountains. Bodhi always felt different and only saw me as beautiful. Yet, I'd still spend a random night shedding tears and feeling sorry for myself.

I didn't like that a few sulking moments of defeat would still pop up, especially since Dip was elevating my life to all time levels. I think a lot of my frustrations stemmed from Goldie. I was tired of her and just wanted to get away. She harassed my dogs constantly. She was out-of-control hyper and had zero discipline. She may have only been a little under 2 years old, but she was an asshole. I guess I couldn't blame her because my parents let her get away with everything. She reminded me of one of those bratty kids that moms let run around screaming and playing on tables in the restaurants. I finally had enough. I had got dumped with taking care of her for twelve months.

I began to suspect that maybe my inflammation with her was amplified because of holding on to so much of my past. I was obviously mad at where I ended up in my life both physically and mentally. That wasn't her fault. I knew I had to dig deep down inside to find out why I continually felt lost and stuck, or else I was always going to be a slave to struggle. No matter how much money I made, or didn't, or where I was located, I was never going to be happy. I had to face the truth of what really fulfilled me and why I kept settling.

One evening, I looked over towards Dip and saw him smiling, as always, while deep in dreamland. Then I looked back at Bodhi to see him staring at me in curiosity. As a few salty drops drizzled down my cheeks, I told him how sorry I was for letting him down. I told him how sorry I was for not having any money for us to move. I told him how sorry I was for adopting him with no secure plan. He looked at me and said, "*You're all we have. We will make it together.*" That kind of faith could never be explained. He knew we'd always be okay. I kissed his sweet little face, cupped his moist snout, and told him how much I loved him. Then I turned out the lights.

I woke up the next morning and things were back to the usual awesome vibe. The snuggles and belly rubs had to be put on hold because Dip had made it through another night without peeing. That meant I had about sixty seconds to get him outside. Like all sunrises, it was about him. Lola snuck up from under the covers and leaped off the bed to greet him with a tail wag and a sniff. Bodhi sprung down and gave him the broskie head lift. We said our good mornings, opened the door to see a welcoming Goldie, and stepped off the deck for another amazing 24-hour experience. No matter the yesterday, it was a new day, and another chance to make greatness happen.

As I watched all of them enjoy their morning routine, I thought to myself, "What a dream come true I'm living!" I had three amazing kids who got more amazing every day... and made life more amazing for me. After twenty-one years of living without my dad, my air was finally coming back. Dip had given me a new outlook. I was gradually reconnecting with ambition, intent, and reason. I knew that if I could help elevate and extend the quality of his life, that I could do it for many more senior animals as well. I could even do it for myself.

I didn't have a target point yet, but I was okay with that. I still had plans for us, and would continue to pursue them to some degree. I just didn't focus on them. Things would work out when they would. The skies were opening up for me and my entire fur family. Where we would go next wouldn't matter... as long as we were together. My Soular System was finally complete.

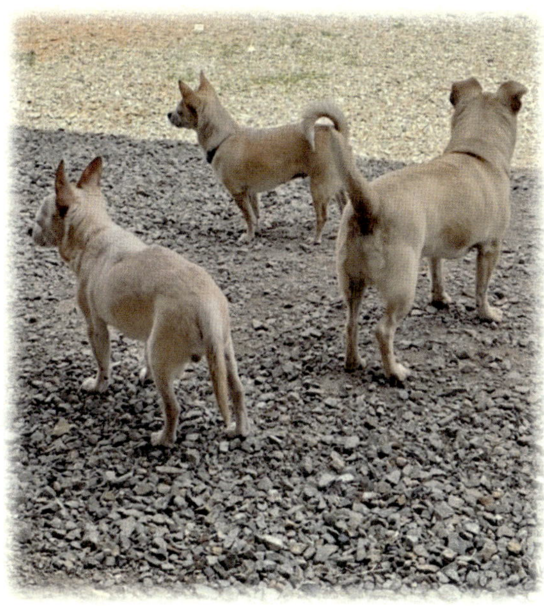

PART 3

Transition
Transformation
Transcension

9
One Day They're Fine, The Next They're Gone

How quickly March became April, then May, June, July, and now we were finishing up the last days of August. Time had flown by. And although I knew better not to look too far ahead, Christmas had begun to show up on my horizon. I was beginning to set my eyes on spending the holidays with my fur family in our own place, possibly back in Los Angeles. Right then and there though, it was all about being present in that super special moment. We were just two weeks away from celebrating our 6-month anniversary with Dip and one fruitful day from him turning lucky 19!!! Things were finally falling into place as the 8th planetary rotation had been Dipper "Veteran" Moon's best month yet!

He was eating great, staying hydrated, sleeping deep, not wetting the bed or coughing, and was exploring and playing outside like the rest of the bad asses. His immunity had heightened to a beautiful level of mental freedom. He cuddled closer and rolled over so I could rub his tummy, and would dig his head under his blankies. He took drives with me to the city, went to auditions, and partially jumped down a few of the steps. His silky fur grew back everywhere, the crusties on his nose disappeared, his nails thickened, and his bones stopped cracking. He no longer had a puffy tummy, his poop was solid, and his digestion had stabilized. Aside from a few times the first month, he never tilted his head again or lost his balance. He still leaned into my hands when I rubbed the side of his ears, and we still sat together while the fresh breeze blew through his pores. Every single day I could see the zest and vitality in his eyes by the way he'd stare into mine. My little boy had beaten the odds and continued to show us the true meaning of inspiration. He had flourished so much that we knew we'd have him for at least another three years!

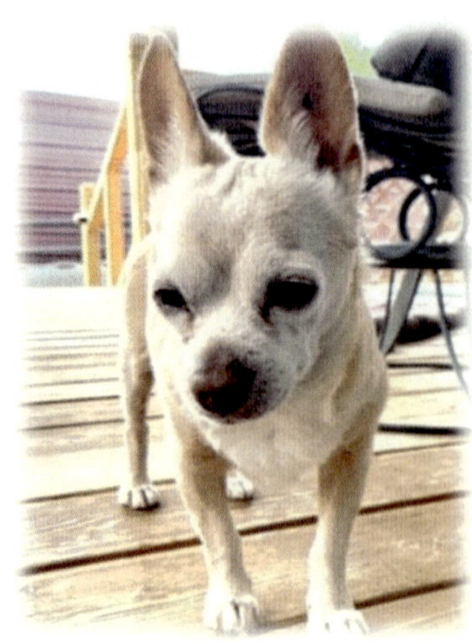

It was a Thursday morning around 7:30am when I woke up to surprisingly see that Dip wasn't up yet. He was comfortably snoozing in one of the deepest sleeps I had ever seen. Usually, the room was dark with the air filter's blue power button as the only hint of light. That morning, the sun had set at a later position and was peaking in through the sides of the blinds. It was beautiful, because a single ray of sunshine was glistening on the tips of his frosty colored eyelashes while he was lost in his dream realm. I was always used to jumping out of bed instantaneously to get him outside to pee. I figured since he was still passed out, I could meditate a bit and spend some extra quality time with Bodhi, and even Lola.

I snuggled Bodes close, cupped his little moist nose, and let him roll over so that I could rub his chest for another ten minutes. I always told him what a good boy he was, how handsome he was, and asked him if he slept well. He'd always respond with some overly excited tail wagging. Then, out of the lower corner of the bed, we'd see Lola peek her head from under the comforter. Her hormones had somewhat settled down in the five months since her spay operation, and she acquired a bit more spark to her step. She'd even let Bodhi do his morning sniff, flirt, and frisk before grunting that she had enough. It was nice when she'd put down her werewolf costume. It would allow us a short window to enjoy the softer side of her.

Bodhi had packed on another three pounds, so picking him up off the bed came with some effort. Lola even gained some girth herself. I guess you could've said that my dogs loved to eat. Even "Vet" filled out his lanky skin and bones so healthily that the rest of his system fell into a perceived balanced state. I was a bit worried about Bodhi though, because I didn't want him to get so plump that he'd develop heart issues or any other health ailments. He went from no rolls at the adoption, to two roles three months later, to looking like a hint of Shar Pei. Maybe he'd been abandoned in those mountains with his brother much longer than anybody knew, and was at the brink of starvation when I met him. He certainly seemed to function amazingly at almost twice his weight.

I was only feeding my kids twice a day and that included top-tier nutrition and vitamins. The problem was that Bodhi and Lola weren't keeping active. It was impossible to take small dogs for a walk in that area without getting attacked. Plus, a month earlier, my stepdad had decided to free up his outdoor senior, so that he could enjoy the last stages of his life like we had offered Dipper. That meant we couldn't stroll over to his side anymore to roam and get exercise. Huevos was an old man and seemed to have outgrown the fighter in him. But I couldn't take a chance that he'd maul any of my dogs. Since my time consisted of Dip on a 24-hour basis, Lola and Bodes weren't getting their workouts. Lola and Goldie still chased the few cars along the fenceline, but Bodhi just wanted to be next to me. I was quickly refueled with daydreams of leaving, and getting to a moist place where we could go on daily treks in soft grass and on sidewalks.

I decided to let the dogs out so that Dip and I could begin our usual morning ritual. It was a quieter forecast. I knew Dip couldn't hear, but I still tip-toed through the hardwood flooring so that I wouldn't wake him. I couldn't wait for his beautiful eyes to open wide so that I could cuddle his little face and body with my nose like I always did. When I leaned in to give him a kiss, I noticed a huge mosquito perched on his snout. We had been infested with those harassing little villains and I was concerned that they'd possibly cause disease in my dogs. Something began penetrating my stomach. I knew seeing that bloodsucker sitting on Dip's nose was a terrible omen.

I fanned the gnat away as quietly and softly as I could without waking him up. Then I sat there for a minute wondering why that day started out like that. Sure enough, within a few minutes, Dip opened his eyes. I said to him, "Good morning, Bobo" (as I also referred to him in that name). "Did you get a good night's sleep?"

He slowly got up, scoped the area out, then nodded, *"Yes,"* and leaned into my face.

I dug my nose into his fur and cuddled all eight pounds of his awesomeness. Like always, I told him how much I loved him and that I was ready to have another amazing day with him. He seemed a little off par that morning, but that was him. Dip would have tons of amazing days and amazing mornings. Then, out of nowhere, he'd have a not-so amazing day or morning. Despite how optimal he may have felt earlier, he was that unpredictable. The only thing I knew, for certain, was that he'd come back around to his vibrant self in no time.

He moped on over to the front door, took in his usual views, and then stepped onto his new "Día De Los Muertos" fluffy mat. I had purchased the cushion a week prior in hopes that it would soften his landing when jumping down the 5-inch step onto the outside wooden floor. Of course, it was blue. That's what attracted me to it in the first place. When I noticed that the little painted skeleton faces were doggies, I thought it was adorable. I had always known "The Day of the Dead" to represent the fun part of Halloween. Oddly enough, it also represented death. It wasn't until I laid it down that got a bad feeling. I even told myself that maybe I should've gotten Dip something else. Being that cemeteries had become prevalent in my recent past, I wanted nothing to do with them, especially for him. I figured I'd pick up a different cushion in the next couple of days, but not until after spending the entire weekend celebrating his birthday.

Dip wasn't up for hanging out like his usual self, but I figured he was just hungry. He had passed out early the night before and then overslept. I had learned that he couldn't go more than five hours without eating. I let him chill out on the porch while I headed into the kitchen to create his morning entrée. As always, he scarfed it up. That was a good sign. From his previous patterns, as long as he still had his appetite, and stayed hydrated, then I knew he was going to be okay.

We reminisced together outside for a bit and then he decided to go back into the house to take a nap. He had a resting system that correlated with how he was feeling. I had recently purchased a smaller doggy bed for him to hang out with me in the kitchen while I'd do some writing. He always seemed to be waiting for me to finish, so I figured I'd keep him even closer. I never wanted him to feel like I was too busy for him. He dug his little anatomy into that bed for about ten minutes, then got up and headed into the room for his favorite blue and green blankets. He laid his little head in first and passed out for the next couple of hours. When he was sick, he could do that. Otherwise, he'd be up every so often to urinate, or to check up on me. Therefore, I wasn't worried.

I was sitting five feet away working through years of notes and ideas when, all of a sudden, he began hacking. I rushed into the room to comfort him and relax his respiratory system. The manner of cough wasn't anything I had heard before. It mimicked the rasping he was experiencing when I first met him in the shelter, but even worse. He had gone through a few bouts of deep, arduous coughs in the past, but in addition to this one, he was also struggling to breathe. His poor little tummy was working hard to accompany his lungs. It was like he was straining to get oxygen. His heart rate was also on fire. I stood him upright in his bed in hopes that it would help clear his air pathway, but the coarseness didn't stop. Then he began dry heaving. I pulled his little plastic bowl next to his mouth so that he could throw up the acidic liquid from his stomach. I always hated seeing him in that kind of discomfort. I was just hoping that it would quickly pass.

Yet, Dip would go on to have a terrible rest of the afternoon. He threw up the frothy mucus four more times, had diarrhea, was lethargic, and didn't have any interest in drinking water. He'd fall in and out of sleep, but I knew he wasn't fully relaxed. His air purifier was on the highest level, and I had his air conditioner and fan running non-stop to keep him at a healthy temperature. By 4pm, he got up from his bed and walked a few feet forward before sprawling out on the rug. The mat was positioned halfway in my room and halfway in the kitchen. I stopped what I was doing, put everything down, and laid on the floor with him.

Was that his last day, I thought? I didn't want it to be. It was less than 24-hours until his birthday and I had so many festivities planned for the weekend. I had gone through similar sequences with him in the 5 ½ months he was with us, but they always turned out to be a bluff. Every one of those times, I'd usually be devasted. Surprisingly, I was accepting and calm. I knew he didn't feel well. The last thing I wanted was for him to suffer in any way.

I had no idea how dogs died, so I made sure to just be there with him fully while doing what I could to comfort every part of his being. Dip's heart rate was extremely elevated, his chest and stomach were pumping in and out, his tongue was slathered over the outside of his mouth, and his eyes were partially opened. Somehow, he was able to fall into a soothing state despite all of the discomfort. Or maybe, he was just too weak to do anything else. My sweet little Bodhi even laid close to him in silence for another hour. He was that empathic and in tuned with what was going on. The Heart and Third Eye chakras were always on point with my little soul child.

Like clockwork, Dip was somewhat back to himself by dinner time. He loved his organic ground-up chicken or beef, and especially adored steak. His herbal vitamins and powder tasted just as yummy, so there was rarely any hesitation in gorging his entire plate. It was good to see him feeling better. He still had that awful cough, but it didn't seem to bother him as much as it did earlier. Plus, he was trotting around the place with some spunk.

I felt I had mastered those "off" days, primarily because we had acquired such a great sense of each other's faculties. But really, who truly masters anything? If anybody had been thrown a fork in the road during the most content of times, it was me. I just knew that Dip had sporadic rotations like that periodically. Sometimes, it would just take a span of diarrhea and a morning of napping for him to feel better. He'd usually be ready to eat and play anywhere between noon and three. If he really had an extra tough bout, then he'd take a full day. So, I didn't think anything of it. I especially didn't feel like it was critical enough to call the veterinarian. Most of the past experiences with her had him suffering severe side effects. So, she would be a last resort, if needed at all.

Dip surprisingly slept pretty well that night and it gave me a feeling of relief. Like us humans, that was his time to rejuvenate. He seemed to be back on track and up with the sunrise like his usual self. It was 6am and time for the celebration to begin! All the dogs jumped off the bed and Goldie came into the room to wish him a happy 19th birthday! They gave him sniffies and kissies and tried their best to play with him in his bed. Dip was acting too cool for school. He knew a numbered label wasn't anything to glorify. To be honest, it was far more special to me. Dip was just ready to begin the day like he knew how. He appeared to be feeling better and wasn't going to wait around for a pack of fools to act silly over another increment in age.

I had to be in the metro city that morning for an appointment, so the plans I made for us would have to wait until we got back to the ranch. We spent a good time outside that morning. I wanted to make sure that Dipper stuck to his normal routine. He was a creature of habit and felt better when he could grasp what was going on. As we were sitting on the bricks in front of the staircase, a gigantic black fuzzy caterpillar crawled next to my foot. He was super groovy! I had never seen a black caterpillar before, much less as huge and furry. Usually, they came to me in white and, usually, they came as my dad. So, I looked it up and it was a Woolly Bear. It was as if he was gracing our presence with his spiritual messages before transitioning into a butterfly looking tiger moth. Butterflies were another one of my insect spirit totems. Therefore, I knew transition was upon us, and was sure that it had something to do with benefiting Dipper!

Maybe I was also going to come out ahead in my case and be somewhat compensated for what I lost. Maybe I was going to be blessed with the means to provide a place of my own for my pets. Maybe I was going to book the audition Dip and I went on together, and finally make it onto a list of actors who'd be guaranteed a job forever. Maybe my mom was going to get her hearing back, be able to retire, and her and my stepdad's dreams of building new houses would come true. Maybe I was finally going to fully regain my self-esteem, and feel so solid, that I could make it through anything. That caterpillar fueled my insides with so many promising outlooks. I knew exciting changes were about to take place... for all of us!

I took a few pics and vids of Dip and then got everyone fed before we drove off. He still coughed along the way. But luckily, we were only there for thirty minutes. I knew he wasn't back a 100%, so I didn't mind if the party had to be postponed for another day. I just wanted him to be able to enjoy it. I had purchased gifts and decorations the previous month, and my mom had picked up a carrot cake for him to safely engulf that Saturday. We also bought him some special raw food delicacies. My mom surprised me with homemade stew meat the night before to carry him through the weekend. We had planned for a 3-day jamboree so, at some point, we were going to celebrate. I wanted his special day to be as special as we could make it together.

When we arrived back to the ranch, the dogs were going berserk. It was like everyone knew the dedicated significance those 24-hours were for Dip. The first thing we did was take our walk through the patches of grass, weeds, dirt, and gravel. Then we went inside so that I could reward the whole crew with pieces of simmered beef. I don't think I had ever seen Dipper that focused. He scarfed down that herbed steak in seconds. I usually monitored his feeding amounts because I didn't want to burden any of his organs. But how could I resist a little overindulging? I knew, that if I didn't stop giving Dip pieces of that stew, he would have eaten himself to the grave. It reminded me so much of my little Charly. I knew that she and Tippet had channeled their love into that monumental moment with Dipper. It was more than apparent in his aura, his energy, and his liveliness, especially after overcoming one of his harshest afternoons. My little boy had made it to his 89th - 92nd doggy year and we were ecstatic!

I had been keeping a progress journal every day since adopting Dip. My intent was to get an idea of what routines, regimens, and treatments could help him improve the most and what would keep him comfortable. He was doing so well in that month that I didn't log as much or take as many pictures or videos. Some of the photos and recordings I did get of him would turn out to be some of his best and most hilarious. The guy could barely walk the first 24-hours after bringing him home. In just eight days, he was running, playing, barking, growling, and taking over the entire castle. By August, he was jumping off curbs and had gotten strong enough to hurdle over the

7-inch barricade that my stepdad placed on his front gate to keep Lola from sneaking underneath. I also caught him crawling under the rakes, and then under the carport, to get to another part of the yard. He'd sniff new plants and weeds, get absorbed in the tall patches of grass, ate dirt, marked his spots, snarled at my stepdad's sweetheart dog, Selina, and always trotted the entire way back to the trailer. I absolutely loved how his galloping back legs exuded his confidence. That strut of his was magical, as was everything he did.

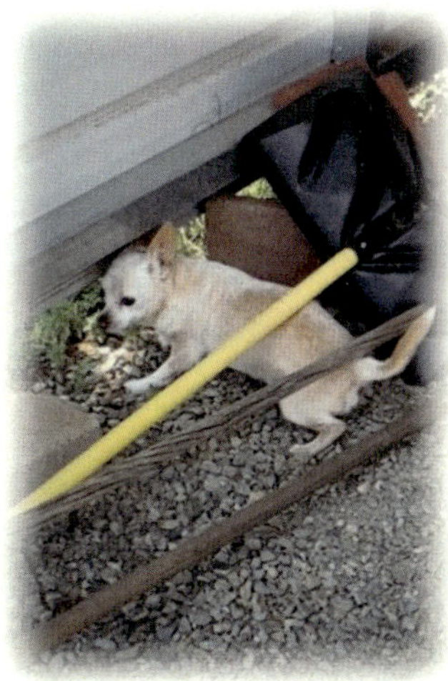

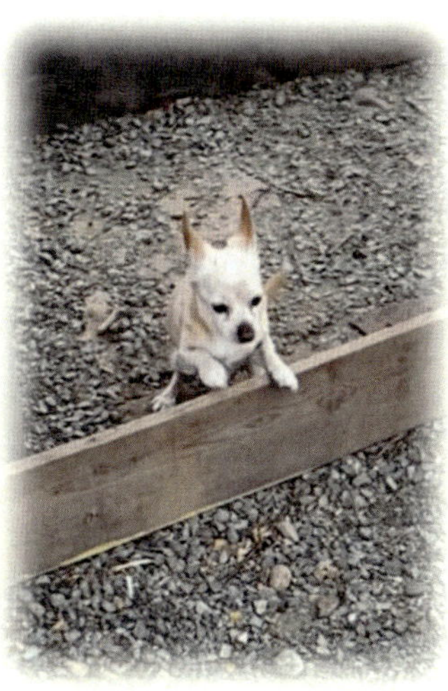

The more Dip came into his own, the more my other dogs did as well. If he could do it, why couldn't they? We called it, *"The Dipper Effect."* If you were lucky enough to spend any time in his presence, you'd become better. He had that innate power just by being himself. I especially began to see it with Bodhi. He had caught on to Lola's ongoing yapping and decided to fully express his vocal cords as well. He whined and howled and barked, and then wheezed because he was so heavy. Then he'd whine again to let you know how much he loved and missed you. Plus, he was always up for what you were eating. He was irresistibly cute and, like Dipper, realized that my stepdad was the weakest link in our family for not being able to hold back treats. He had developed dignity and, for sure, privacy... as he never took a shit in front of anybody. Yet, he had no qualms with walking into the bathroom while I was doing the same thing.

He also didn't take into account that I was laying next to him every night when he'd free float some gas balls in his sleep. I was praying that Goldie wasn't rubbing off on him. I couldn't imagine his ass smelling like hers. Yet, by the next morning, he'd act like nothing ever happened. He'd venture through the yard and find his way up to the fence for a standoff with my stepdad's 80-pound senior canine. As cute as it was, it gave me a bad vibe. If Huevos got out, he'd probably take Bodhi's life. I kept a close eye on him when we were outside and let him battle Goldie instead. No matter how tough Bodhi thought he was, he never lost an ounce of his precious, calm disposition. He even found a way to hold onto my hands so that I wouldn't stop rubbing him. His tail was a giveaway, as he'd wag it for almost anything. Then he'd follow me like a shadow and stay just as close as Dip did.

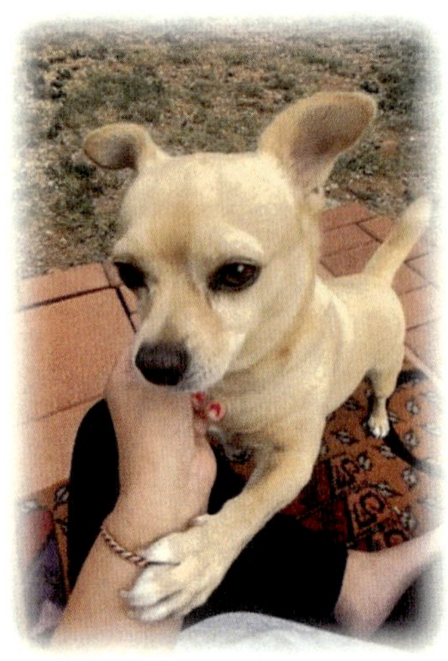

As for Lola, she surprisingly developed into a much nicer dog. I still wasn't fully connected to her, but I was pretty sure that her hormones were at a level where Dip wasn't in any more danger. She had become Loli Boloni, Lola Ventrana, Bonita, and the baddest chick on the planet according to all other members of the household. She was also gaining some ranking in the most annoying. I'd have to yell at that dog twenty-five times a day for barking at absolutely everything. She'd sit on her outdoor cushion and yelp at air for hours. Then she'd come in the house and give my stepdad some ear lobe and facial cleanses.

On the early morning weekends, my mom would head outside to walk 10,000 steps around the property. She'd opt to take Lola and Bodhi so that they could get some exercise. That lasted about twenty seconds. Lola would fall over and refuse to go any further unless you dragged her. Obviously, nobody had ever taken her on daily tours. It was hilarious watching what a little diva she was. Like always, Bodhi just went with the flow. He knew he'd get a yummy bone afterwards as an incentive; totally defeating the purpose. The dogs had been so spoiled with bones that if a forensic tv show ever came to investigate, they'd probably be able to put together a full skeleton. Yikes!!!

It was interesting how Bodhi and Lola could be so different and, yet, be such great friends. Maybe opposites did attract, or maybe Bodhi was just that easygoing. Whatever the formula, it was working. Those two would sometimes share beds, give each other kissies, and gang up on Goldie. Then Goldie would wait until I was out of the picture so that she could go after Lola and roll her. I was finding myself even more upset with that dog. She just knew how to ruin the mood. That was probably the reason Lola never fully shed her mean girl skin. She wasn't ever vicious towards Bodhi, but I still had to watch her. He didn't know better and I didn't want him to get his face bitten off. She didn't know how to conceptualize anything playfully. We thought maybe her behavior was due to her previous owners abusing her. We were rooting for her, but only time would tell.

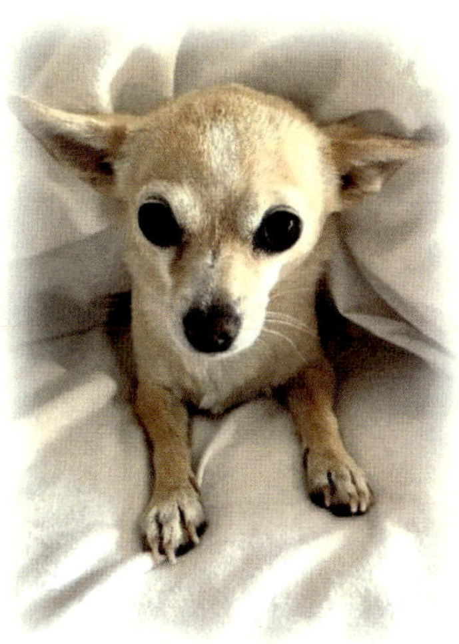

Bodhi turned out to be the smartest of them all. While Lola was too busy spewing venom at Goldie, Bodhi was getting cuddles and kissies. While Lola and Goldie were chasing cars along the fenceline, Bodhi was receiving treats in the kitchen. While Goldie was testing Lola's patience, Bodhi was enjoying chest rubs on the cushions. They were dumb and he knew how to take full advantage of it. In addition, he always gave Dipper the first of everything. He was that unselfish.

I knew Dip appreciated the companionship from all the dogs, including annoying Goldie. I couldn't have been more grateful for the kind energy they shared with him. I watched how they protected him and stayed close. They also gave him his space. He'd have an agenda as simple as standing still in the 12" strands of grass for two minutes not doing anything, and they'd still crowd around absorbing his electricity. Anywhere he'd walk, sniff, mark, or shit... those dogs would think it was as amazing as fried cheese. Whatever he did, the collective enthusiasm heightened.

Although I'd become a bit defunct of establishing a bond with Lola for how she initially treated him, Dipper didn't hold on to any of it. I was the one with the sour taste in my mouth. I had kept a grip on the emotions attached to those few incidents. Yet, they'd be hanging out in the yard as if nothing ever happened. It was like, *"Yesterday's business doesn't serve a positive purpose."* If only I could've let go of past mishaps like he did, and allowed myself to be free of the heavy, unnecessary energy. My dogs were wise souls. They had the type of instincts that would take mankind lifetimes to learn.

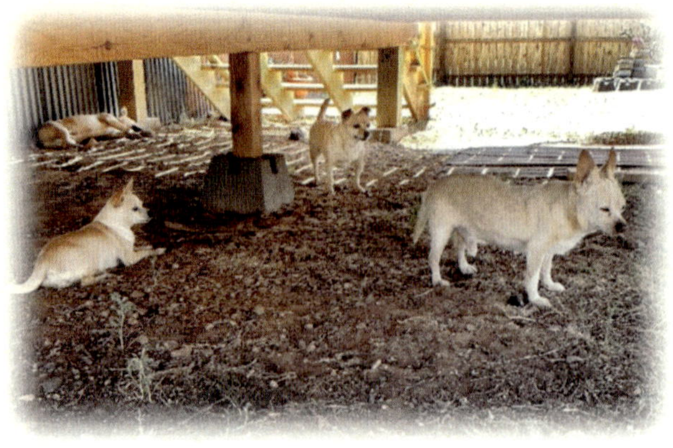

It was Saturday and Dip still had his cough, but it didn't seem to be wrecking his entire day like that previous Thursday. I monitored his heartbeats and constantly checked his tummy to make sure he wasn't labored in his breathing. Everything seemed like it lessened and he appeared to be okay. We spent most of the day fooling around on the property and taking plenty of breaks for some more yummy stew treats. That round, something was different. Dipper couldn't catch his front footing while eating. It was as if he was so zoned in on the food that he couldn't hold himself up. He'd slide open wide onto the floor to lick up any leftover shreds. I thought it was so cute. My little darling looked more and more like a puppy. I knew I was doing a great job. To see him enjoying those party favors made me proud.

It was evening time and Dip had a delicious cake awaiting him. We sat him on the sofa, lit the mini fireworks, and brought in the desert while singing Happy Birthday. He didn't have any idea what was going on. All he could do was concentrate on that frosting. It was one of the funniest kodak moments of his existence. My mom grabbed my phone and I picked him up so we could make our wishes together. I told him, *"how much we loved him – how much we couldn't wait to spend many more with him – may that one be his best one yet – and may everything come to him in optimal health and love and companionship and friendship and markings and stinkers!!!"* Then we blew out the candles together. Once I removed the fire, Dip attacked!

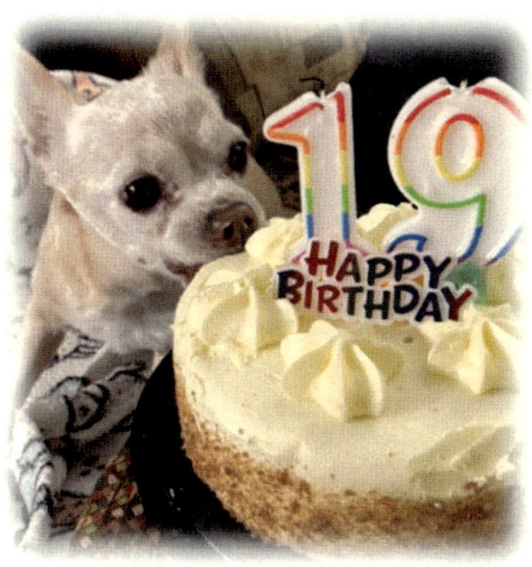

What a rewarding feeling it was to be a part of making an impossible, possible. Words couldn't describe how thankful I was for being in a position to make that little boy's life so jubilant. I had been granted one last chance to finally get it right… and I got it right. In fact, I had been getting it right: from Charly and Tippet, to Bodhi and Lola, to my beautiful little Dipper. I would never be okay that it took Fritz, Peaches, and my beloved Rudy to suffer, for me to learn how important the entirety of a pet's life was. Because of them, I became a better human. In turn, their light helped give my dogs better lives.

The Universe was sending all sorts of signs that weekend. Dip recovering was the most important one. He certainly seemed to have bounced back. By Monday morning, things started out a bit slowly, but I credited it to the Holiday hangover. He took a few steps towards the entrance and I noticed a difference in his ambiance. He was almost pure white just like an angel with a furry halo circling his Crown chakra. I could envision a white lotus atop of his head connecting to the heavens. He was standing in the front doorway gazing into the day's elements when, strangely, tears appeared. I didn't know if they were happy drops from being so grateful, or sorrow drips from knowing something I didn't. He stood there for a few minutes and then closed his beautiful lids. I stayed there thinking that I could stare at him forever. He was that beautiful. He was that meaningful.

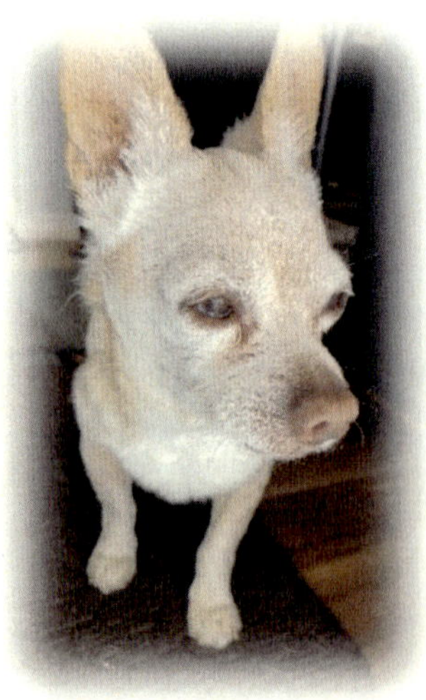 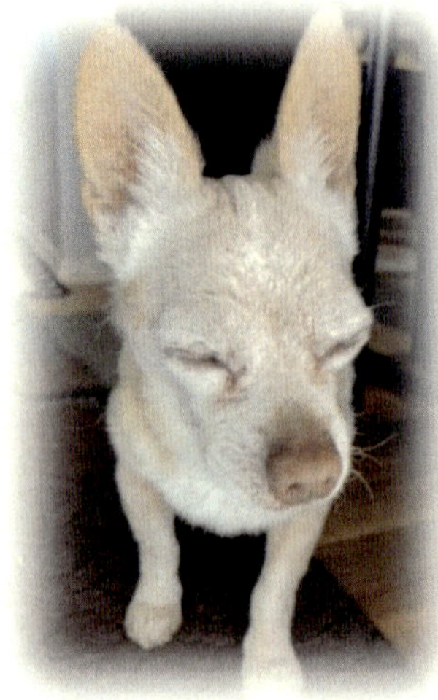

Something was unique about that day. It wasn't as hot as it had been, and the air was comfortable enough to stay outside longer than we were used to that summer. Mosquitos usually didn't come out as much in the fiery sun, so Dip spent a good portion of time getting lost in the tall grass. Just as I was sitting on the front step watching him, a tidal wave of emotions surged within my gut. I had no idea where those feelings were stemming from, but I was about to gush my eyes out. I was highly in tuned with my digestive tract and knew that something was coming to an end... again. Yet, I felt it to be golden. It had to be. I had just seen a fuzzy black Wolly Bear caterpillar!

For some reason, I went back to my legal matter. I had received an email from my attorney the previous week in regard to a potential settlement meeting by mid-September. It would be a "9" month and the closing of the lunar summer. Since "9" meant completion, then maybe fate was falling into place so that I'd finally be freed of that past experience. There was a possibility that it would be over. I thought that it must've been what was triggering me. I gathered my composure and smiled through the tightness in my stomach. I didn't want Dip to have anything to do with those proceedings.

I walked over to where he was hanging out under the carport, and noticed him facing forward with an interesting stance. I'd seen him in a familiar pose when he was drawn to the light in the hallway, so I figured his spirit guides decided to connect with him outside as well. His tail was upright, which was a good representation of a healthy pancreas; at least it was in his case. As I was watching him hold his place and focus, I forgot about my tears.

Like earlier that morning, I just wanted to sit there and stare at him. Then, he actually began to turn around. I was completely shocked because Dipper never turned back. As quickly as I thought he'd make that move, he stopped in midmotion. It was as if he was thinking of telling me something, then realized that he couldn't. He never fully swiveled his neck and head, or looked anywhere behind him. He didn't even look in our direction. After a minute or so, he returned to his forward position, took two steps towards the sunlight, and walked to the other side of the parking garage. My intuition told me that he was about to enter an even grander phase with us.

My mom got home later that evening and I told her how emotional I was all day. She was aware of the recent epiphanies and felt that maybe they were happening the last few days of August, so that I could spend September closing out that horrible chapter. Then I'd be able to enter the "1" month of October (10 → 1+0=1) with a fresh start. I realized that maybe Dipper hadn't been feeling as well because he was also helping to purify my system. We were a combined unit. Being as connected as him and I were, there was no doubt he could channel my senses, as I could his. I just didn't want him to have to go through any distress due to something he never had anything to do with. Thankfully, he was feeling better, so the last of the release would solely be on me.

Later that evening, one last cosmic signal would pay me a visit. It was after 10pm and the whole crew was outside roaming the land. Dip and I were on one of our last pee walks for the night. I looked into the midnight blue sky to see if the Little Dipper was out yet, but it wasn't. I don't know what made me think of it, but I wondered what I'd wish for if I saw a shooting star. Not but a few seconds later, a sparkling comet shot over the back of the mountaintop. I couldn't believe my luck! I instantly wished to win something in my legal case, because I knew it would benefit all of us. From the signs, the emotional day, and all the insect totems… something big was coming!

Unfortunately, I woke up at 4am that Tuesday morning to Dipper hacking profusely. I checked his heart and it was pounding. I knew I had to get him outside so that he could let off some steam. He had a few squirting poopies, so that told me he wasn't feeling well again. I thought maybe I'd take him in to see the doctor later that morning to make sure it didn't get worse. Just as I was waiting with a baby wipe to clean his tender little butt, the sparkling Little Dipper showed up. It was perfect timing. We went back inside, took a few walks through the hallway, and then he settled back in his blue and green blankies.

Dip got back up before my mom went to work at 6am. By then, he seemed like his usual playful self. He went outside, took another poop, and then came inside to take a run through the hallway. My mom and I were so glad to see him doing his usual morning runs, but then he started coughing. We were used to him running out of steam, so we didn't think anything of it. The weird thing was that I had already made four trips to the bathroom that morning. I didn't have anything to drink since 8pm the night before. My mom left and, almost immediately, Dip could barely move. He had his head lifted up and was slightly stretching his neck back as if trying to breathe. I hopped into the shower and placed him on the bathroom rug. When I peeked out, he couldn't hold himself up. I instantly got out, picked him up, and left a voice message with the vet. When they opened, they called back to tell me to bring him in right away. I began to think that maybe I was channeling his little body and urinating the fluid out of his lungs, since it appeared that he was too weak to do it himself.

As I was getting ready, I could see my little boy progressively deteriorating. He wasn't coughing anymore, but was moving in slow motion with his neck still lifted and stretched out. I hated seeing him that way, and something told me that it was probably going to be his last day. He didn't eat anything and continued to move in a daze. I placed him in his bed, in his favorite blankies, and stuck his Mookaite and Blue Calcite crystals underneath. We said goodbye to the dogs, not knowing if Dip would be coming back. Then I loaded him into my vehicle. The heaviness of sadness permeated my nervous system.

I kept my right hand on him the entire drive. His neck was lifted and his mind was floating into outer space. I'll never forget the way he was looking at me. I knew he was telling me it was time to go.

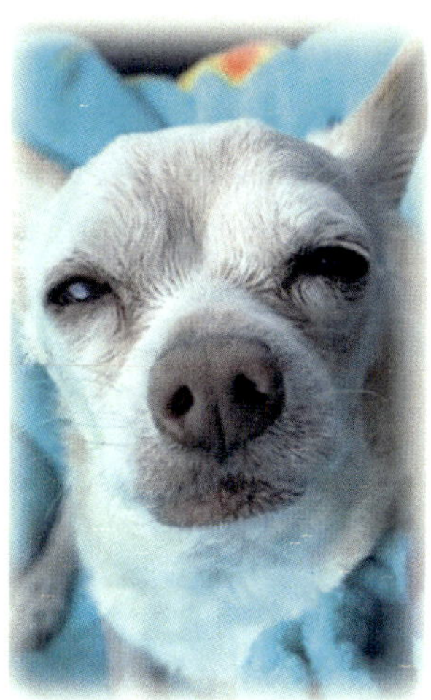

I rushed him into the animal clinic as gently as possible. They came in, took his temp, and he seemed to be okay... for the moment. His numbers looked fine, so they took him back to get the first ever x-ray of his chest. While they had Dip in the radiation room, the doc came in and told me that she thought he had pneumonia. She had already injected him with an antibiotic and a potent liquid diuretic without my consent, or even knowing his prognosis. I was furious!!! I knew Dipper couldn't handle any medication, much less protocol dosages. The meds she had prescribed in the past were so harsh on him. Before she could guess at anything else, one of the assistants brought Dip back in. She said that he *heard* my voice and became too nervous to continue. I took him into my arms and, of course, he relaxed.

By then, his stomach x-rays came back showing that he had eaten rocks. I informed the doctor that Dip would eat dirt and that was probably how the microscopic pellets got into his belly. I figured that must've been what the problem was. She wanted to keep him for a few more hours while they waited for his blood results, and heart and chest x-rays. I had planned to take Dip with me to the metro city that day so that I could get a haircut. I figured I'd have enough time to get in and out of the salon before picking him back up.

With the previous lockdowns, and that year of living with my folks in the mountains, my hair had grown to the bottom of my back. There were so many other amazing aspects to share with Dipper that my hair didn't matter. I also hadn't kept in contact with anybody, except those closest to me. My life had changed so much that I wasn't interested in the same things anymore. I didn't care about makeup, fashion, premieres, golfing, playing tennis, casinos, or traveling. In fact, one of my friends had contacted me in early August asking to scoop me up for a 3-day vacay to Miami. Four years earlier, I would've jumped at the opportunity. But I had Dipper. I didn't want to miss a single second of his life. Getting a haircut was the closest to being social in two years.

The trip only took an hour drive and my appointment another hour. Just as I was starting my truck, the vet called to say that Dipper's x-rays came back with an overflow of fluid in his lungs. They had him on oxygen for the time being, but he would have to be administered a large dose of the prescribed heart medication and diuretic for the rest of his life, and immediately beginning by the time I got him home. I told her that I wasn't giving Dip anymore of the meds that almost killed him. I explained how he had increasingly flourished with homeopathic treatments, acupuncture, laser therapy, organic food, and non-synthetic vitamins. I let her know that I wasn't a vet. But based on seeing how toxic those drugs were, it would be fatal for him.

Her response was, "If you don't give him both of those medications tonight, he's going to die." Then she followed with, "Have we discussed euthanasia?"

My life was slipping away in a matter of a 5-minute phone call. Actually, my dog's was. He was just fine yesterday. And now, I didn't know what was happening.

I submitted and asked her, "How long would we have to wait before they took effect?"

She replied, "I already injected him with another dose, and then it would be another couple of days for his heart rate to go down."

I was sick to my stomach. I should've never left him to go get my hair cut. I raced back and met my mom at the clinic. When they brought Dip into the room, he looked like an entirely different dog. He was more youthful and radiant than I had ever seen him. Sadly, I knew that meant him and I were going to have to change our routine. My amazing mother paid the outrageous bill and we headed home.

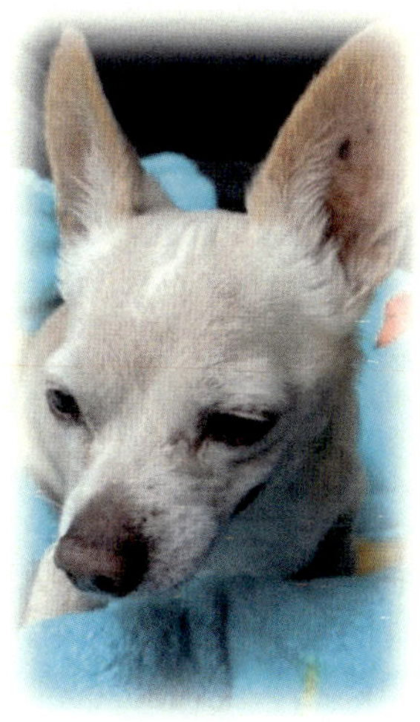

He didn't want to sit in his bed. Instead, he wanted to sit on my lap like always. I cushioned his sweet fragile body with his Heart chakra green blankie and we made the 45-minute drive home. By the time we reached the underpass, I thought maybe he'd feel up for a roll down of the window so that he could take his usual inhale of the mountain atmosphere. I went to lift him up, but he was too weak. He sat back in my lap and tucked his head into my stomach.

By the time we got home, all the dogs were excited to see that Dipper made it back. We were all excited that Dipper made it back. We got out of the truck and Dip walked over to one of his favorite pee spots. He looked like he was doing fine, but I could tell that he was beginning to move like a zombie. That was no surprise. I had just got done telling the veterinarian that very thing. I thought maybe if he ate, he'd get some of his energy back. He hadn't consumed anything all day and had been injected with a double dose of a medical diuretic, as well as an antibiotic for pneumonia that never showed up in his blood tests or x-rays. I let him do his thing while I unloaded his bed. Then I went inside to cook some ground-up organic meat and steam some veggies.

My mom brought Dip in and I could tell he was ready for some good grub. I placed a hearty sized serving in his bowl, but just couldn't bring myself to give him that pill. He was pacing the kitchen, knowing that I had been cooking, and was looking at me with those adorable eyeballs. I peeled my fingers from the countertop and grabbed a knife to chop the tablet into powder. I almost threw up in his hamburger meat. I didn't want to give him the drug, but I held my breath and crumbled it up into his saucer. It would be the very last time in my life that I would go against my gut.

It was obvious how hungry he was by the way he initially tore into his food. But with about a quarter of it left, he backed off. He'd do that every so often when he just wasn't feeling it anymore. Yet, I could see that he was beginning to lose his balance. I thought maybe it was because I still had to give him the other part of the prescribed cocktail. So, I filled up the tincture and did the best to squirt the liquid into the sides of his gums. I hated every second of giving him that medication. I could immediately tell that it was just too much for him.

I took him outside to walk around and pee out what he could. I sat on my usual bottom step of the front staircase and let him wander off. He only went a couple feet further. Not but a few minutes later, Dip collapsed. He lost all movement of his body and neck. I instantly scooped up his paralyzed little frame into my arms. He was turning blue, his tongue fell out of the side of his jaw, and his eyes were rolling from left to right. Then he began choking and gasping for air. I laid him on his back and rocked him like a baby, as I paced around in front of the carport thinking that would supply him with more oxygen. My mom was walking over from my stepdad's and I screamed out that he was dying!!! His soul was leaving his body and it was shattering!!!

What was so harrowing, was watching my baby cry out in pain while looking at me in complete fright like, *"Why is this happening to me?"* I told him that it was okay for him to go as I rubbed his tummy and head as softly as I ever had. I, too, couldn't understand why he was being tortured. I then walked him up to the porch deck so we could sit on the outside patio swing in hopes that it would help calm his sympathetic nervous system and yin meridians (lungs, heart, stomach, pericardium, spleen, kidneys, and liver). We stayed outside as the dark sky covered the magenta sunset, and I held my little boy in my arms, close to my chest... while he slowly suffocated.

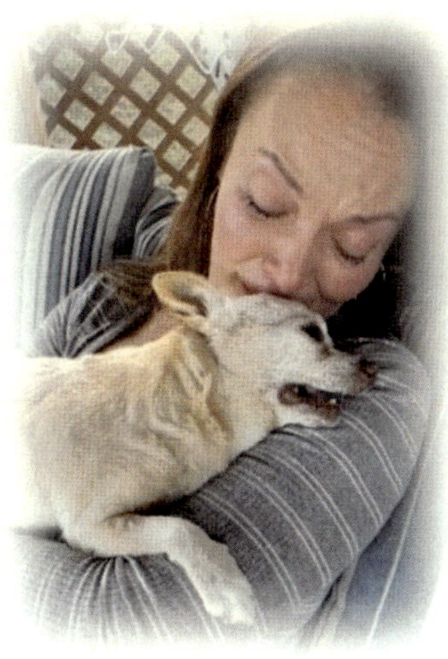

I finally took Dipper inside as it was getting even more dreary. He seemed to have calmed down. But really, he had already died in my arms two or three times. Just when I thought he would take his last breath, thirty seconds later, he would come back to life. I sat with him on the couch bawling my eyes out and holding him as gently and close to me as possible. I delicately comforted every part of his body. He was helpless and exhausted. As much as I didn't want to lose him, I just wanted him to go quickly so that he wouldn't have to suffer any longer. As I laid there numb and blurred, Dip took one last long stretch, and then his final breath. I felt his little body fall into his skin and onto the left side of my clavicle. I knew he had left the earth. I tried to check his abdomen for a pulse one last time, but there was none. My little boy was gone.

I walked down the hall with him and, as I passed the wall mirror, I saw him dead on my shoulder. His eyes and mouth were open and his tongue was sprawled out. Death was so unkind and ghastly. I had never seen it as up-close or as acutely. It would become a haunting vision forever engraved in my mind. My sweet little Dipper was lifeless and still looking at me.

I laid with him in my mom's room for another couple of hours and cried and cried, and told him how much I loved him. His little corpse was damp from my liquid pain droplets trickling down my cheeks and onto him. I never wanted the sun to come up again. I just wanted to fall into his same sleep and disintegrate into stardust together.

I realized that my mom was going to need to come in and call it a night at some point. I got up and walked Dip down the same long hallway that we would walk through ten times a day to get our exercise... the same one we'd run and play up and down in... and the same one he'd walk towards the light in. I carried him into my bedroom and laid his little departed body onto his favorite blue and green blankets. I shut his eyes, put his tongue back into his mouth, and gently closed his jaw. I placed his bed on top of my mine and, for the next eight hours, I sat there rubbing his cool silky fur, his big beautiful ears, and his collapsed Third Eye. I held his paws like I always did and told him how much I already missed him.

By morning time, he had stiffened and cooled. It was awful to watch the expiration process unfold. I padded up his pretty little face with the layered blankets and put him in the passenger seat right next to me. It would be our very last drive together. We wouldn't be sticking our heads out of the window and breathing in that mountain air. Instead, we'd be hand in paw the entire ride into town without a single bit of motion or sound.

When we walked into the clinic, there was only one assistant present. She was my favorite, actually. Thank goodness she was the only one in attendance. I wasn't prepared to let that doctor know what I thought of her. She looked at me with the brightest of smiles thinking Dipper was just back for a checkup. Once she saw my bloodshot eyes, and the pain behind my facemask, her cheeks fell to the floor. She became overflowed with liquid sadness. I didn't speak a single word. I handed her Dip and his bed and walked out the door. That was the last time I ever saw him in that form.

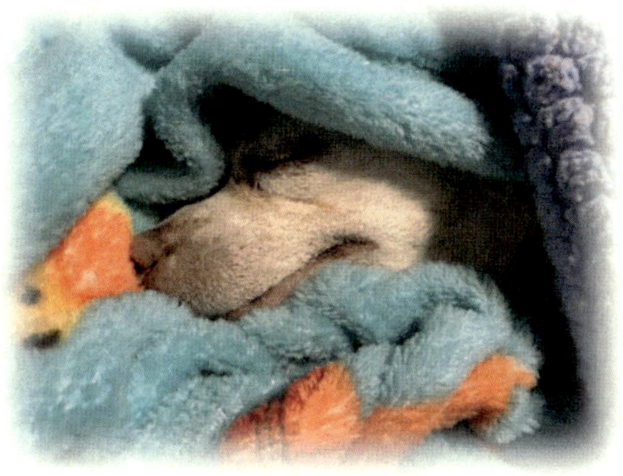

10
The End of the World... in Stages

It was the morning of September 1st and a day dedicated to celebrating the existence of my amazing dad. Although it had been twenty-one years without him in physical form, we still carried on the tradition in memory of his beautiful spirit. Never in my past did I associate completeness of the "9th" month with a negative context. I had always seen that first day as the onset of something spectacular. It was my dad's birthday; how could it not be? So really, the only ending was the closeout of summer for the emergence of autumn's colors. My annual ritual usually meant spending that day reminiscing down memory lane with my original best friend, my soulmate, my everything. Instead, I was submerged in the longest drive of my life after dropping off my dead dog's body.

There were no errands I could run or anything I could pick up. In fact, I couldn't even stand up. I got in my car and headed straight back. As I traveled that lonely road home, I cried more than I had ever cried before. It made me wonder how my body could produce so many tears. Trust that if I could have wept myself into my own death, I would have. I couldn't even lift my arms to wipe my eyes because my muscles felt so heavy. From turning the steering wheel, to getting out of my vehicle, to opening the gate, to parking under the carport... I hurt. It felt like I had an ice pick in my heart and pancreas. Actually, it was like the mini ax was perforated in all of my organs, and I was bleeding through my punctured wounds. I slightly lifted my eyelids to see the property eerily deserted. There were no excited dogs jumping around to greet me and no lovable Dipper to unload out of the car so he could take his usual stroll. He was nowhere and everything was somber. I quickly sensed a gravitational force gluing me to the gravel pathway. It was as if anxiety was keeping me from having to walk over the exact spot where he helplessly collapsed.

I opened the door and stepped into the trailer only to find Bodhi excitedly awaiting to kiss my eyeballs and jump up on my shoulders. Lola was just as enamored, but kept her distance so that she wouldn't get stampeded. Goldie wasn't present, so I figured she was over at my stepdad's. My dogs were always used to me coming home with goodies, and showering them with love and expressions of how much I missed them. The gusto quickly faded when they saw my pale, hunched over self about to fall to the floor. Plus, there was no Dipper. I felt so bad that I couldn't reciprocate the same kind of energy, but I was inconsolable. I couldn't breathe, I couldn't see straight, and I couldn't communicate. I dropped my keys on the counter, kicked my shoes off, and staggered towards my room like the ghost of Gloom.

Two of Dipper's beds were sprawled across the floor in an L-shape around the corner, but were frigid and vacant. He wasn't napping in them or playing under his covers or sitting there figuring out how to scratch his ears. He was back at the clinic, dead, laying in his favorite third. I couldn't explain the pain of seeing the empty space where he inhabited such peace. I could literally see an outline of his furry figure sleeping in beautiful comfort. When he'd wake up, we'd spend time staring into each other's eyes and then we'd snuggle and rub our ears, chins and noses together before the rest of the crew tried to join in.

It was a dreadful feeling. The loneliness echoed and all I could see were those haunting visuals of his last moments. Complete shock and sadness were understatements. I was also covered in mosquito bites from my stomach to the inside of my groin, and the length of my legs down to my toes. I had been wearing thin leggings, flip flops, and a half shirt while going through the whole ordeal. The last thing I was concerned about was me. Instead, I thought I'd have him longer and that we'd have another year together. But I was wrong. It was the first day of completeness and all I could think of was that my life was over.

Just as I was about to crash into my bed, Lola sat on her hind legs and waved her arms to tell me that she wanted to go outside. Somehow, I back peddled far enough to let her out and then made my way back to Bodhi. I picked him up and we crawled under the covers together. The weather was in the high 80's. Yet, I was freezing cold. I just wanted to cower into my cave and decompose.

I didn't know how long I laid there, but it felt like an eternity. It was as if I was six feet deep laying in my open casket waiting for dirt to bury me. Then I needed to pee. I looked over to Bodhi and his warm-hearted stare asked me if I needed help walking to the bathroom. I did, but I didn't want to burden his gentle soul with the weight of my sorrow. I peeled myself out of bed and made my way towards that famous hallway. Of course, he followed me. I couldn't inch but two steps before almost throwing up and breaking down into hysterics. That hallway was Dipper's red carpet. It was a magical ride in the simplest of forms and the avenue of our daily rituals. Absolutely everything was a reminder of him: every room, every pattern, every door, every smell, everything. It was all so empty. I don't know how I made it to the toilet, as it seemed miles away and I was crawling at night without my flashlight. Really though, it was only eleven-thirty in the morning.

I sat there long after urinating just trying to feel my fingertips. I was so numb and mentally disjointed that I don't even remember wiping. I know, it sounds gross, but that's where I was in that moment. I do, however, remember washing up afterwards. As I was drying my hands, Bodhi was standing there with an odd look on his face. He knew Dipper was gone; he could feel that loss. But it was as if he was trying to tell me something. I crouched down to cup his little moist nose, but tears were pouring down my face and onto his. I rubbed the side of his ears instead. That's when something tenderly uncanny happened. He leaned into my hands and fell into them the way Dip used to. He almost dropped to the floor like those same leaves in the autumn that were Dipper's signature season. Bodhi had never done that before. That wasn't his trademark move whatsoever. At that exact second, I knew Dipper was with me.

It was a weird mix of sensations because, although he came to me, he still wasn't there physically. I had only been without him in bodily form for some hours, so I wasn't in a place where I could fully appreciate communication from the other side. All I could do was try to hold my stomach lining in as I kept gagging. I was also selfish and just wanted him back in person. I knew that I'd get there someday, and the sign definitely gave me the faith I hopelessly needed.

Before Bodhi and I reached the kitchen, my mind completely shifted. I was in absolute shock and couldn't think straight. But after that sign, I realized that I couldn't let death take over the aroma and feel of our home. I was pissed that Dipper was taken away from me, but I didn't want to smell the decay, the gases that bloated his body, or the liquids that were draining from his mouth by the next morning. I didn't want to feel the chilling stiffness of his limpness or the touch of his unresponsiveness. I didn't want to hear the anguish of his torturous transition. And I certainly didn't want to see the fear in his eyes in those last minutes of his life. Rigor Mortis was not what Dipper represented.

He was so much more than those last hours. From his beautiful essence to the nucleus of his beingness, he made every aspect of our living space wondrous. Why would I want to remember him in any other form than the pure love we shared every single moment together? I was completely heartbroken and knew that I had a tough battle ahead. I also knew that I had to purify the energy around me so that I wouldn't drown in despair. My intent was to bring back a lighter atmosphere. I didn't know if I could do it, but I was going to try. It was the only strength I could muster up. I knew that the way to start would be by clearing my space of all distractions.

Within minutes, it was like I gained bionic powers and instantly began a tornado of cleaning. It was as if I was functioning as a machine and, for the next day and a half, I didn't feel anything. I took apart my bedding, linen, clothing, rugs, dog blankets, dog beds, and even derailed my vehicle. I vacuumed every crevice of the house and car, did laundry, dusted, washed countertops, dishes, the bathroom, and took down all solo pictures that were taken of me during my past relationship. In a flash, I reverted back to not understanding the timing of anything. So, I also decided to pack up my crystals, statues, Zen animals, and art. I even packed away my vision boards and all other spiritual symbols that were known to manifest optimal love, health, and abundance. I didn't want anything in my room that was the slightest bit of encouragement, because none of it had worked for shit. Barely any of those affirmations came true and all they did was remind me of the wishes and plans I had for me and Dipper.

When it came to social media, I got off those platforms. Aside from my fan page and *Furever Soulmates*, I was rarely on them anyway. They had become monopolies flooded with separation, algorithms, political and health propaganda, and censorship. They also leaked people's personal info. I was lucky for the respect, class, and kindness that most interested visitors offered to my pages, especially with all the global hatred. I just couldn't communicate on any level with anybody. I permanently closed personal channels, pages and profiles, and deactivated my main and public networking forums.

As difficult as it was, I also decided to put *Furever Soulmates* on hold. I had gained an immense amount of life-saving knowledge from Dipper. I learned gentler and more natural ways to heal and care for dogs. Our experience together became so meaningful that I wanted to do more for seniors on every level. I knew I could promote holistic and homeopathic treatments, and share stories as ways to extend the quality of life for all pets. Yet, I just didn't have the same willpower. Nor, could I see poor abandoned doggies in desperate need for forever homes. I had to set it aside while I grieved.

Amazingly, there were so many others out there already doing the same thing, and even more. There were tons of people and pages and causes and organizations who made it their 24/7 life missions to save seniors. They were also getting homeless, abandoned, and abused animals off the streets and out of awful situations. They were fighting for animal rights, getting laws changed, finding innovative ways to heal and improve, disarming cruel practices, and teaching awareness of a pet's importance. They weren't going to slow down because I wasn't posting anything.

I felt content with walking away temporarily so that I could cope and do my best to recover. I knew I'd return at some point, and was sure that everything would pick up just like I had left it yesterday. That was how amazing the world of animal lovers and rescuers was, and one of the few bright sides of the internet. It was also because people had been just as kind to my *Furever Soulmates* pages. I was blessed to have that type of following when so much of the web was filled with horrible energy. Clearly, it was evident how low the earth's human inhabitants were vibrating. I didn't need any of it.

As drastic as the world was changing, it did bring me an answer I had been desperately searching for during the last half of my stay in LA. I had gone back and forth whether or not to remain in the entertainment business. The times I thought I was done, I'd always get sucked back in. I had been away from that scene for quite some time. And because of Dipper, I found myself enjoying other things. My goals with him were constantly changing. I still found myself slightly hanging on to that last thread of acting. But once vaccine mandates took effect, I wasn't allowed to be hired for most projects. Whether I'd ever give it another shot in the future, I was done for the time.

I terminated my local contract and didn't attend another audition again. My second to last was with Dip, so there was no better way to go out. As for my agreement with my primary agent, I felt it would also eventually dissolve. She was on the same page as me, but knew that it would be some time before things changed; time that I didn't have to waste anymore. Both reps were honest, well-respected, quality driven women. It was an honor for them to believe in me, and my talent, enough to submit me over the years. Upon our closing, my local agent told me that the doors would always stay open. I knew my other agent would do the same. They were both that genuine.

Without question, I felt defeated. But not necessarily due to my career shifting. I knew that ship had sailed long ago. I was more relieved than I was disheartened. The only hope I lost... was for life. I started looking at it as if I was shedding myself of even more, so that I'd leave even less to deal with after I was gone. I didn't want to go on. I just wanted to die. The way everything was playing out, it looked like it was falling into place. Was it my destiny, or was I creating it all based on what I learned from spiritual philosophy? In that instance, neither. That's why I packed up my stuff and quit praying to air. I was so bitter at a supposed higher source for putting Dipper through pain and agony, that I knew I was finally done. I had struggled with the belief of a certain form of upper guidance my entire life, but that final act closed the coffin. What I didn't realize, was that I had already begun my travels through the nine islands of death. And in each one, I'd have to confront myself. It had been the loneliest forty-eight hours of my life. In that time, I had quit the world, God, and Facebook.

After everything was said and done, I was sitting in a spotless room with bare walls. I was just waiting for Dipper's favorite bed, his blue and green blankies, and his ashes. Surprisingly, I wasn't attached to that soot. I couldn't see him in any form other than his eight pounds of awesomeness. I still wanted them, but I didn't feel the same energy through them. I decided to design my own urn and fill it with some of his crystals, pictures, and sentiments. I took a quick trip into town and found a cool little wooden box with a beautiful clasp. It was perfect. I decided to keep his large Blue Calcite heart crystal and two of his smaller Mookaite stones that used to comfort his emotional body and immune system. I placed the heart on the empty space where Dipper use to sleep and the Mookaites on top of my dresser. I was still flushing stress out, so I had to go to the restroom. When I returned, my dear little Bodhi was keeping Dip safe and protected. We all missed him and we all mourned for him. My parents and the rest of our fur family were now minus one Moon, and we knew that life would never be the same without him.

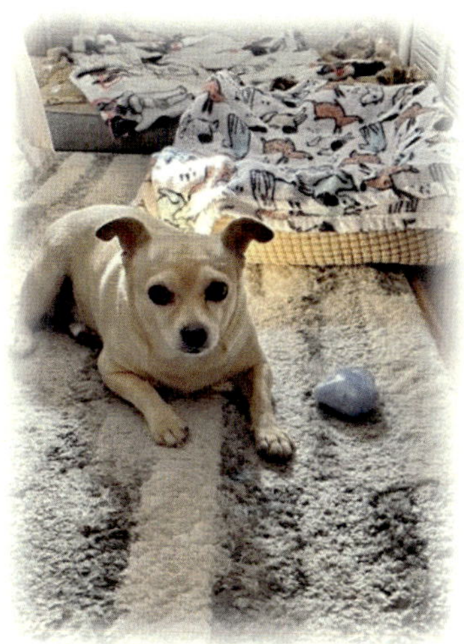

By the end of that second sun and moon shift, I was actually able to doze off. I hadn't slept in almost two days, so my body was exhausted. I prayed that Dipper would come into my dreams, but he never showed up. That stretch of time sure was a blinded haze. It also turned into something cathartic.

It was the third morning of the month… the third day without Dipper… and the beginning of my third published book. The ambush of emotions had reignited and I literally couldn't breathe. There were no words to describe the physical pain I was in. But somehow, I managed to open up my laptop and begin typing my sadness. My mind had always worked in different ways, so it was no surprise that I could do something like that at such an excruciating time. I had nothing else. Writing had been my savior my entire life. It was the best therapy in the world for me. I wish I could've said that I consciously chose to start on that day, but I didn't. That day picked me. The number "3" had always brought harmony, wisdom, success, and vitality to me. It would be no wonder that I would begin writing about my 3rd little Moon on that 24-hour rotation. I didn't have any clue how it would go. I didn't even know if it would go at all. I pretty much couldn't lift my fingers. I just knew it was what I needed in trying to come to some kind of understanding with why my dog died.

I spent quite a few hours letting my emotions come out on the pages. Nothing was organized and I didn't have a projected design or format in mind. It was more like one long journal entry. I couldn't speak any words to anyone, so it was the only way to express how I felt. The more I wrote, the more I realized that I was right back at the starting point of six stages of loss and death that I knew all too well. They had become a pattern of continual coping mechanisms throughout my adulthood. Apparently, I hadn't done a good job of getting through all of them by the way I progressively got worse with each depletion and hardship. It looked like the shitty process was starting all over. And once again, I was beginning another dreadful trip of my life.

I learned to make do as a young adult and found that the process of loss undoubtedly begins with shock. There are people and pets with terminal illnesses, and once favorable relationships, jobs, and leases that we know are coming to an end. Still, are we ever completely prepared for the day we finally lose them? Add unexpected departures to the equation, and how can anyone react in any other way than shockingly? It's a harsh inner stun, that's for sure. But we are sentient beings. We start and finish where we do, and when we do. In the middle is where we grow. The layers can shift just as erradict as the winds transform the climate, and the energy can spiral into another phase as it did with me. Although my little boy came to me through Bodhi, the anger I developed became overwhelming.

I was already pissed off at God. I couldn't accept how the supposed creator of a loving, gentle, fragile little creature had caused that same being so much pain on his way out. Dipper didn't deserve that. Then almost immediately, I had extreme disdain for the veterinarian that killed him. I told her that he would die if I gave him those drugs and explained how he couldn't handle medication, much less the dosages she was prescribing. She had no interest in what I had to say about observational therapy or the debilitating side effects that drugs had previously caused him. Then she had the nerve to ask me if we had discussed euthanasia. She had given up on him so quicky. How dare her. How dare her take my dog's life so lightly.

I was also furious at the owners who had the audacity to surrender him to a shelter. How could they put a dog that age through such emotional trauma? How could they not have the compassion to find him a loving home, instead of sticking him in a cage to die? I was just as livid at the volunteer for being so rude to him and the shelter for neutering and vaccinating him. I was pissed at Bodhi and Lola for attacking him that first day, and even more pissed at Lola for being so mean to him that first month. I was upset at where my life had ended up and, how I was so stuck, that I couldn't move us to a grassier, more humid environment. From the simplest of things like my stepdad telling me to wait until he stopped eating one day and started going downhill, to my mom placing him in the middle of the living room when I was gone, to the various social media sites not giving him an ounce of attention... I was angry.

In a sense, it felt like some sort of blame game. I was mad at everyone and everything, and unbelievably hurt that it ended the way it did. As quickly as shock extended into resentment, guilt entered the station. That's when fault got placed on yours truly. The "would've, could've, should've," and "if only." I began tearing myself apart for leaving him at the shelter after meeting him, then waiting six days to adopt him. Even worse, was waiting two weeks to meet him after coming across his photo, knowing that he'd be mine. Maybe I could've voiced my concern enough to prevent him from acquiring a shitty cough and undergoing unnecessary surgeries and vaccinations.

I raised it a notch and tore myself apart for discontinuing his acupuncture and laser treatments a month earlier because he had excelled to unheard levels. I figured he was doing so well that I'd give him a break and let his system work its own magic. Since we didn't have to come into town for the appointments, that also meant the cement walks at my mom's office stopped. He absolutely loved those. On top of that, I wasn't taking him outside to play as much as he was used to. The climate was reaching extremely hot temps and I couldn't take a chance of overheating his system. Plus, it was mosquito season, and I had to do what I could to keep those bloodsuckers from eating him. We even stopped taking our usual strolls on my stepdad's side because he had given his larger dog the freedom to live the rest of his life outside of his enclosed yard. All three of my pups were appetizer size for him, so that was no longer an option.

Dip loved the outdoors more than ever. Yet, I kept him inside an air-conditioned bedroom with a filter blowing out boredom. To make matters worse, I also decided to dive back into some of my writing projects in hopes of bringing in an income again. I had so many plans for us and knew that my books could potentially offer an opening to those avenues. I'd be at the kitchen table working on my laptop. He'd be laying in his bed just staring at me with the anticipation of, *"When can it be just you and me again?"* How dare me.

Several thoughts came up as to what I could've done differently and how I could've done more. My brain was convoluted with self-criticism. How could it not be? He was a 100% dependent on me and my responsibility. I let him down and I let him die. All I could do was reflect back to those last moments that I had with him and how I ditched him. I absolutely hated myself for leaving him at the clinic for three hours to go get my hair cut. Who would've known that we would only have a short time left? Then, the vividness of that phone call in the salon parking lot stabbed my cerebral cortex like the same ice pick in my heart and pancreas.

Aside from being adamant that drugs were the only way he could be helped, she thought I'd consider putting him down. I remembered thinking, "What the fuck is happening?!!!" Then, after discarding that idea, she actually had me believing that drugs were the only way to save him. Obviously, that turned out not to be the case. Not only had I decreased his exercise, and one of the vital means at helping to flush fluid from his lungs, but I also gave him the medication that killed him. Talk about a pitchfork through the chest cavity. I may not have realized to what extent the lessening of walks had on him, but I knew better about the drugs. My gut told me that I was making the biggest mistake of my life, and my heart just wanted to extend his.

I don't think anybody who experiences some form of tragedy can undergo a series of shock, anger, and guilt without being tied to grief and sadness. I was devastated. Dipper was my everything. And since he'd been gone, I had nothing. There was no longer a copilot venturing into the city with, no best friend to play and take walks with, no more being inspired daily, no soulmate to communicate with me cosmically, no furry partner to snuggle nose, chins, and ears with, and no more Moon to share unconditional love with. I just missed his baby soft smell and the brilliance of his pupils.

I couldn't bring myself to go outside or sit on our favorite bottom step to absorb the sun and cool breeze. Two feet in front was where Dip's soul began its exit. I couldn't even walk on the same brick setting or gravel pathway. I avoided everything that reminded me of our routine and didn't dare let the dogs walk over the empty space where his bed used to lay. I had even created cool emergency cards for each of my dogs with directions on how to take care of them in case something happened. Dipper's section was especially eye-catching. Anybody who came across that card wouldn't have had a problem in keeping him alive and well. That was my intent, but it was no longer needed. On top of that, I had to remove his microchip info from the website because he was deceased. Checking that box was tough.

It made me realize that sorrow was the core generator that linked every stage of death. It wasn't going anywhere no matter how each level of emotion preluded the next. I was heartbroken through the first four, there was no doubt about that. But now, I was also lost and empty, and felt like a failure. I had become dependent on money for everything, barely owned any belongings, and had little to show for my hard work in my adult life. Talk about feeling like a waste. How could I see the silver linings in anything? How could I have faith and direction for a future that had melancholy written all over it? Add to that, nothing having the same meaning anymore. I started to find my way, my vision, and my tenacity when Dip was with me. Since he was gone, they were gone... and I was lost again. I had nothing in sight but dying. That's where the compilation of sadness became dangerous.

Feeling so low, hallow, and broken-hearted made appreciating the present moment almost impossible. That was Dip's most significant characteristic and I felt powerless. I knew it was all I had, but it was difficult to weed out the painful distractions when impulses were a roller coaster of intervals. One day I'd feel slightly better than the previous. And others, I felt worse than ever before.

I remember taking a drive into town one morning for my first acupuncture session since his passing. A vision came over me of suddenly swerving my steering wheel so that I'd veer off and crash my car into the side of the mountain. Never had I contemplated hurting myself in any way, so those unfamiliar thoughts scared me. I knew I didn't have the guts to take those graphics seriously, but something told me I needed help.

Maybe it was because I'd been without my independence for so long and yearned for a quiet space of my own. I needed to work through the process, but there was rarely time for just Dip and I. I was still living with my parents where the talking was constant, let alone their annoying dog. I seldom had pure silence. Not only did my world suck, but I couldn't stop reliving Dip's death. It didn't look like I'd ever recover. I was doomed, and certain that I wouldn't make it to the aftermath. The dark setting brought me back to a parallel time, twenty-one years earlier, when my dad died.

It had been almost two weeks and, although I was somewhat eating and sleeping, my body began to ache in places I never thought could ache. I was glum that time had already passed so quickly without Dip. I knew that if I didn't force myself to move around, I was going to continue a treacherous path. That's when the guilt of getting better set in. It took me to the moment when I returned to Los Angeles after my dad's funeral and spending weeks packing up his house. I had no idea where I'd go from there. But fortunately, I lived alone and had all the quiet space in the world to journey through my mental hemisphere. There was a book waiting for me and it was called, "Tuesdays with Morrie."

I had heard about the piece a few months before my dad passed and it caught my interest. I had understood the story to revolve around a professor and a student, and how their reconnection brought about substantial life lessons. It was a book about friendship, mentorship, and how each could help the other remember what was truly important. I had only been in LA for a little over a year and everything seemed to be skyrocketing for me. I just wanted to make sure that I was centered with what really made me happy.

At that time in my life, that paperback was the first reading I dove into after my dad was cremated. I cried through every line as it reminded me of the wisdom and light in his soul. It definitely touched on areas of my path and career, but more on letting go. From there on, I began the 17-year-journey that it took for me to grieve and cope. I thought that maybe it could help me with my current journey since the circumstances were similar. Dipper died on a Tuesday and of the same complications as my father. He also died a day before my dad's birthday. Maybe I was looking too deep into it, but I felt it in my gut. That was one thing I was never going to go against again. Like all the signs in my life, those pages came to me in order to help elevate. I knew I was being brought back to re-read them for a reason.

I began the book on a Tuesday morning and by the late afternoon, I had finished. It didn't quite have the same meaning for me the second round, but the characters and backdrop surrounding my current loss were different. What it did give me, was a moment of serenity. I did a sitting silent meditation for another hour, and then joined my parents and my dogs to enjoy what I could of dinner and a movie. My mood was monotone, but at least I wasn't bawling my eyes out and choking on pity. It was the first evening we spent together as a family without Dip, and I made it. I smiled and even shared a few laughs. I hated that he wasn't there with us, but I made it.

By ten-thirty, Bodhi, Lola, and I were already deep in sleep. I hadn't remembered a single dream since Dipper died, whereas I used to recall them like I was shooting live on a tv or film set. I became a slumber slab of deactivation and just prayed that I would get enough rest to help my body rejuvenate. In the middle of the night, I faintly heard Bodhi gasp and then sigh as he exhaled. I paused for a few seconds to listen for his next breath, but it never came. I wasn't sure if it was some form of PTSD that I had developed from Dip's final moments, so I panicked. The room was almost pitch black and all I could see was a limp silhouette. I checked for a heartbeat and felt nothing. Then I lifted one of his paws to see if he'd wake up, and it dropped. I shouted out, "BODHI!" and began shaking his chest. Before I knew it, the dude sent me a savage growl for interrupting his dream.

I thought to myself, "What is going on with me?" I had already been having premonitions of my stepdad's previously combative 80-pound rescue dog escaping through the gate and killing him. We had spent almost a year hanging out on that side before Huevos was freed to live out his best life. Although he had become a sweet dog in his older age, you could still feel the tension between him and Bodhi. They were the only two males left on the property. I didn't trust him or the fence, so I became a hovering parent. Bodhi wasn't allowed to go anywhere near that area without me anymore. My mind had become unstable and I felt like I was a walking time bomb. I had sailed to five of death's islands and just reached the sixth on my floaty boat. Fear was the next of my pathos.

The last thing I ever guided my life with was fear. So, how could I become inundated with it and in the smallest forms? There was no way I was going to let that stage get the best of me. Anxiety wasn't going to rule me like it had tried to in my past nightmares.

Funny enough, that incident with Bodhi accelerated both his and Lola's pampering. Those two owned my bed and had me working as their doggy concierge. I became the servant who was there to provide snuggle blankies and sacrifice my sleeping space. I always wished that Dipper could've enjoyed that same luxury. But I couldn't take a chance that he'd walk off the side and crack his spine. He was fearless. But, at times, he was restless. I provided him with a 5-star hotel suite of bedding and comfort and, from the way he snored, he didn't seem a bit left out. Even though I was in a slump, I was down to two Moons and had to protect them from the same awful thing happening. That previous night was a bit of a wakeup call to try my best and listen closer, attend to needs more, and make sure to be even gentler.

I couldn't have ever seen myself being extra sweet to Lola since we had our previous issues. But the weirdest thing happened. Almost immediately after Dipper died, she latched onto me like a leech. I couldn't get away from her. I actually started having visions that she'd be the last man standing and I'd get stuck with her. I didn't know what it was, but something had shifted with her. She was suddenly mellow, engaging, and playful. Even her tail started wagging and she moved with a pep in her step. It was as if she made a 180-degree turnaround and became an entirely new dog. Then she took an interest in Dipper's beds as if they were an indoor playground. She'd jump in and out of them, roll around, and play under the covers like he did. She'd want to lick my face off, hog Bodhi's sleeping spot next to my pillow, and be as close as she could. The more I hated that she softened up after Dipper was gone, the more she wouldn't leave me alone. Why couldn't she be nice when he was still alive?

I knew it took time for rescues to feel safe, but something told me that maybe Dipper was channeling his love through her like he began to with Bodhi. He had that galactic power when he was on the ground with us, so why wouldn't he have it from up above? Maybe Lola was becoming a true little princess instead of a predator. Maybe she was switching from mean girl to sweet girl. She'd always have multiple personalities, but the nice ones were starting to stick around longer.

It became clear which of her chakras were most activated, and those were her Sacral and Solar Plexus. Just like Charly, she felt every emotion and sensation deeply. But she took it further by touching on both temperament sides of the spectrum. Then, like Tippet, she had a huge bark and intense purpose in her actions. Yet, she also had a confident bite. She was the 2nd of our Moons and represented the fire in alchemy. Her lust with the cushion progressed, she had a love/hate relationship with Goldie, and she didn't hesitate in showing that dynamite could come in small packages.

There was all that hoopla, and now she was friendly. The more I looked at her, the more I saw an innocent doggy who longed to be part of a family. If there was any imbalance in her Manipura, then that was most likely the culprit in why she had control issues. Maybe it was her time to shine like Bodhi and Dipper had begun many months earlier. Maybe she was finally learning how to trust and accept love again. And in doing so, she was taking my attention off the sadness. That little girl may have had her own issues, but maybe she was there to help me move forward by remembering the light that Dipper shared with us... and how he didn't hang on to anything less luminous.

As for Bodhi, no matter how activated his pineal gland was, he still always had a look of fear in his eyes like, *"You're not leaving me, right?"* I knew that being abandoned haunted him, and it was my life's mission to make sure he never got left again. Bodhi knew that things were different since Dipper had passed. I just hoped he understood that it would only be temporary. He saw me cry in anguish and pain every single day and still made sure to lift his paw up so that I could rub his belly. That was our way of telling each other not to worry. As long as we were together, we'd always be okay.

It had been almost three weeks and I hadn't talked to anyone other than my parents, stepbrother, and acupuncturists. My sweet mom and stepdad had been incredibly supportive and left me alone to work through things. Nobody else knew the extent of what I was going through. I don't even think anyone knew that Dipper died. The last photo I posted, or texted, was on the day he turned nineteen. Even though I was making some progress, the pain was still throbbing.

I wanted to be able to rejoice in the memories we made together instead of being stuck in a swampy lagoon of mortality. So, one morning, I told myself that I was going to replace "I miss you" with "I celebrate you." Every time I looked at his pictures on my phone, watched his videos, or just laid down staring at the vacant space where he used to sleep, I made the effort to say, "I celebrate you... I celebrate us." I went from selfishly needing him to appreciating the time I had with him. Unfortunately, that only lasted about twenty-four hours before I was right back to "I miss you" every other sentence.

I had to admit that the "I miss yous" sparked some light into my system. I began thinking that maybe I should finally reach out to those closest to me since some of my friends were starting to get worried. One of my dearests, Deidree, was especially concerned. She had gotten word from my mom almost immediately after Dip died. Not only was she one of my best friends, but she was also my mom's amazing hairdresser. We knew each other so well that she completely understood how I could isolate and withdraw. Still, she sent me the most heartwarming and encouraging voice messages every few days. I never picked up once. If only she knew that her type of love and friendship was one of the major reasons why I kept going.

I was lucky to have friends that shared a special form of togetherness. Another one of my kindred sisters, Alana, was one of the most empathic people I had ever met. Combined with drive, perseverance, and self-determination, she was also one of the most pleasant. I had met her almost four years earlier during the first week I had moved in with my ex-partner. Who would've ever guessed that I'd meet one of my most treasured friends from that piece of work? She was actually the only one he allowed me to see and stay in contact with. So, in the end, the Universe won again.

I watched the hard work, studies, and sacrifice pay off in a professional career she dreamt of. In addition, she worked at evolving more of herself, her personal relationships, and made it a huge part of her life to help improve the welfare of shelter animals. She was a walking inspiration paving roads for up-and-coming young women. We spoke all the time. Yet, she was two weeks from relocating to Texas and hadn't heard a word from me. I felt terrible because I wasn't going to be there to send her off with love and support like I intended. The deal had been a year in the making and I was looking forward to helping her prep for the move and celebrate her last month in town together. I knew she'd been struggling with uprooting and leaving a place she had lived at for over sixteen years, because it meant giving up her independence and all she had established. I knew she needed me more than ever and I just couldn't be there for her. Thankfully, we had developed such a strong bond that, when the air cleared, we'd be able to pick back up like nothing happened.

She was aware that Dipper had died. But like everyone else, I didn't have the strength to speak about it. As with Deidree, she also kept in touch. Every few days I'd get texted some caring words and symbolic emojis. Although I didn't respond, they also helped me. By the time I finally replied, she had already traveled across the state border and had been crying for hours. I took a walk out on the front deck, peered towards the mountaintops, and stood there listening to the birds singing summer's songs. When Dipper was alive, everything sounded so much better. Yet, for a moment, Mother Nature allowed me to be with my friend Alana, and only with her. I had always been blessed with an innate gift to uplift. I was going through one of the most challenging times in my life and I still chose to be fully present. It was sort of like an out-of-body experience. I was able to switch frequencies just like that day when I purified my entire living area only a few hours after seeing Dip for the last time.

When we finished exchanging texts, I continued opening up and did my best to try and reconnect. I knew it would be painful having to send out sad pics and words about that day, but people cared about me. They knew how much he meant to me. If anything, it was the perfect time to say, "I love you and thank you for being so mindful." I explained that I'd be out of contact for some time while I processed it all. Every soul-lighting friend of mine completely understood and were just as compassionate and sympathetic. It was nice to feel the supreme love they shared through memes and a keypad. I especially remember another one of my dearest friends giving me such a beautiful explanation:

"Just a thought, maybe it was such a struggle for him because he desperately wanted to stay with you... meaning his soul. But his body was too worn out and that was what you were experiencing as far as the pain went. How grateful I am for you that you had this amazing unconditional love for the time that you did, and still, so heartbreaking that what you are left with are the memories. You took the time to nourish a relationship and love will live on forever."

—Angela

I was blown away. *"My little boy didn't want to leave me, but he had to. That was the struggle."* Her text, and many others I received from my beautiful parents, Shaian, Nellya, Tim, Fitz, my stepbrother, my acupuncturists, and even one of Dip's homeopathic companies gave me a glimpse of optimism in trudging forward. After hanging up the phone with his veterinarian that last afternoon in the salon parking lot, I sent out an emergency email to one of his primary health and nutrition teams. Their products had been helping to extend his quality of life for over five months. I felt confident with them because of the friendly way they communicated with me. They were always a 100% honest, even if I didn't agree. For some reason, they weren't able to get right back to me that day. I wanted so badly to hear their input, so that I could make an argument as to why I wanted to avoid giving Dipper drugs in those last hours. The incident ended up unfolding the way it did. Yet, once I got to a place where I could start talking about it, they responded. Their letter was just as touching:

> *"I am so sorry you both had to experience his end in that way. Please do not beat yourself up. I am a firm believer that none of us leave before it is our time. It is a shame your last memories were so traumatic, but try not to live in that space, he does not. He is now pure energy enveloped completely in love. He would not want you to focus on the end, but rather on how you opened your home and your heart and made his last months happy ones."*
>
> —*With sympathy, Maria*
> *(The Pet Health and Nutrition Center)*

I was honored to be surrounded by such warmth. It was also nice not to have to hear that "he was old anyway." As empty and lonely and dispirited as my life had become, deep down inside, I knew I wasn't alone. I had a long way to go, but I had my parents first and foremost, my dogs, friends, stepbrother, packed-up crystals, spiritually awakening symbols, and people like them. I had also learned from *Furever Soulmates* that there were millions of other animal lovers out there that had gone through similar experiences. If I just reached out my hand, those that were meant… would connect.

11
The Messengers and Messages

I continued writing what I could in my book, and it was holding parts of me together. Acupuncture was helping as well. Aside from meditation, stretching, writing, nutrition, and a slew of other alternative techniques, integrative therapy had always been a powerful health tool for me. I had a homeopathic team my entire stay in LA and was lucky enough to connect with a few other aligning healers while being back home. I wasn't stretching, working out, eating enough veggies, laughing, earthing, or barely journaling. I had no motivation to do much, so I had to force myself to attend my once-a-week sessions between two different practitioners in two different cities. I loved them and it was the only reason I made any attempt.

One morning, my local specialist noticed that I didn't seem to be getting better and recommended that I see a grief counselor. She wasn't aware of the temporary spans of slight progress I had made. For some reason, every time I'd step into her office, I'd break down uncontrollably. The same went for my other specialist in the metro city. I couldn't open my mouth without exploding into tears.

I sat with my local acupuncturist and we talked about the pain I was going through. She told me that I had always been sad, even before my dog died. I thought to myself, "Of course I was. I had lost everything. Then my dog came into my life and revived me. Then he died. I should be sad." I explained that I had been through loss and death more than enough times in my life, including the passing of my dad. What was bothering me was how Dipper died. He didn't have to go through what he did and I just couldn't grasp it. In so many words, she explained that he had shifted into a different dimension and, like birth, his transition may have appeared to be intensely agonizing. Most likely, his soul had already left his body. He was free and en route to that perfect place of harmony. She asked, "Why would you want to hold him back from achieving that state of being?"

I wasn't with my dad when he closed that final curtain. So, I didn't witness the harrowing act of expiration straight in my face. I was far away, but I didn't feel as helpless as I did with Dipper. The guilt of not being there with my dad until the very end, and not being able to say goodbye, weighed heavily on my soul for half of my life. It also didn't help that I didn't pick up his last phone call.

But I saw my dog collapse and turn into a coil spring. Then he suffered in my arms for another hour gasping. Finally, he took one last stretch and breath before his fallenness set. I was able to be with him, comfort him, and hold him close to me until he left his body. As much as I wouldn't have wanted it any other way, I wish I would've seen the illusion of "goodbye" differently. I was still grateful that I didn't let him die alone. I had to believe that it was the best way for him to go because he was surrounded by my voice, my touch, and all who loved him. I didn't go through that with my dad, so lingering images of his soul leaving his envelope never haunted me. She didn't know anything about what happened with my father and I didn't disclose it. I just told her that I missed my dog more than anything in the world. Then I laid there in silence while she stuck needles all over my body.

I drove back to the ranch after my session was over and all I thought about was how I had to remove my grip. There was no doubt that I was drowning in sorrow, but I was also holding Dipper back from his travels. I was keeping him from experiencing pure love and energy in its entirety. I couldn't do that to him no matter how much I missed him. I didn't want him to have to worry about saving me. I wanted him to bask in whatever form of heaven he was in to the fullest... just like he did in the time he was with us here on the earth's surface.

I pulled onto the property to see Bodhi, Lola, and Goldie eagerly barking for me. How could I be anything less than happy? Fortunately, my stepdad had been so kind to doggy sit every time I had my appointments. I got out of my vehicle, and we shared our normal, exciting routine. Then surprisingly, Bodhi and Lola wanted to chill on my bed with me. As I laid there staring at the ceiling, I knew I had to force myself to celebrate and feel gratitude. I grew sadder every day because I saw him in everything. But how could I not feel pure bliss knowing that he was in a state of euphoria? I had tried the previous week, but knew that I had to be consistent. Teardrops flooded down my face as Bodhi was cuddled up next to me. All of a sudden, Lola crept up from under the covers and, of all the dogs, licked them off. Dipper sure had a way of channeling his love.

I felt like I'd been laying there for hours without a pulse, but then my mom walked in the house and the dogs dashed off. She had picked up Dipper's powdered remains for me. I couldn't bring myself to be anywhere near that veterinarian. A couple of days after Dip died, I had written her a scathing letter lined with harsh criticism. I sealed it and asked my mom to deliver it when his ashes were ready to pick up. Since they took three weeks longer than expected, I was able to calm down enough to revise it into something more in tuned with my kind personality. I still told her that I didn't appreciate how she took my dog's life, but in a less obtrusive way. Surprisingly, my mom told me that she had retired and wasn't even there. Who knew if she'd ever get that letter? Something told me it wouldn't matter. I had a feeling that her guilty conscience got the best of her.

After we finished dinner, I decided to call it an early evening. I'd usually do a silent meditation or an hour of one of my favorite Solfeggios. But I was mentally drained and just wanted to fall into a sleep coma. A wet storm was coming in and the winds were shifting. Thank goodness moisture was upon us. I was looking forward to dozing off into another mind space while rain pellets smashed the rooftop. Then I could sit in my room the following morning while the sprinkles drizzled down the window sills.

The dogs and I held onto our hair and fur, and went outside to take our last bathroom break for the night. As I stepped onto the front deck, I noticed a 4-inch-long bright green leaf stuck to the top of our outdoor blinds. I couldn't figure out how it got there but, more so, how it didn't move when the gusts were so ferocious. Then, all of a sudden, his legs extended out and he began climbing. It looked like he had long thin antennas helping him find his way as he was heading in between the 2x4's for stability. I realized that it was a Moving Leaf, also known as a huge Katydid. I only knew that because I took a picture and sent it to my stepdad. He was a human encyclopedia that knew everything about nature and all of her creatures.

The insect was incredible and one brave mofo. He stood out on our wooden porch like a duck among dolphins, and I wondered why he wasn't camouflaged in the trees. We were a dry dust-colored climate, and the dude was neon green. I had never seen one before. I had only seen a Praying Mantis. In fact, a little stick fella showed up on the screen door a week before. My mind was so fogged that I didn't realize another amazing courier came to visit. I guess our Earth's Mother kept at it so that I'd finally pay attention.

I had always related green with luck, prosperity, and protection. Yet, almost immediately, my Heart chakra popped up. I believed that colors played a role in the spiritual world, and my heart was the center of my compassion, love, and forgiveness. Yet, I couldn't feel any of it for myself. It was in pieces and my energy and wallet were in shambles. Yet, the more I thought about it, the clearer his messages got. I was having difficulty with physical and spiritual equilibrium. I couldn't accept Dipper's new transformation or the beauty of his transition. I was stuck on his bodily form and how tragic he left it.

I had always felt that my lower three chakras represented my physical and material aspects, whereas the top three were more about my spirituality. My heart was the middle core that balanced them. Maybe he came to remind me that each of the seven wheels of energy were still one in the same system no matter their functions or characteristics. That went for Dipper. He was still a part of the whole. No matter his functions or characteristics, he'd still be present.

I was completely wowed, and also ready to get out of the cold. The wind was atrocious. I called the dogs back in just praying that he'd make it through the storm. It looked like he'd be okay because he found a safe spot that blocked the draft. I watched him take shelter and said my goodbyes. Right before calling it a night, I looked into the phenomena a bit more. I wanted to see the metaphysical meanings and timing behind his presence. I began to see more of a link between his anatomy and my story. The long thin antennas, that guided him on the blinds, were sensory receptors. No wonder he didn't seem scared. His intuition, sight, sound, smell, vapors, and awareness were on point. I couldn't help but link those feelers with the human Third Eye. Maybe it was a sign that I had to re-activate mine.

I also noticed that he represented transformation. I wasn't sure what that entailed, but I had entered six stages of my own. Anything involving changing form was a sign that growth and evolution were upon me. By his shape and hue, it seemed like he could blend in with the trees. Yet, he was standing out prominently. It made me think that I had the power to reshape my life and its brightness as well. After watching him adjust, adapt, and maneuver his way to safety, something told me that I'd also be okay... because I could do the same. He stood there motionless until he was ready to make his next move. Why couldn't I be just as patient while going through the healing process? No wonder he came to me when he did.

It was inevitable that things would be different. His guidance was a reminder of what I had known all along: nothing was guaranteed, constant, or permanent... we only had the present moment. It took me back in time when members of the same critter family paid me visits. They always showed up to convince me to take a leap of faith. Usually, they came around when I was considering changing careers or residences. There was no coincidence with the leaf bug. In a way, I had the same inner conflicts, and was in need of the same lessons. The traveling messengers were the only ones that varied. What I loved most about his vital force and wisdom, was that he opened up my heart to strengthen how I would perceive the seen and unseen from then on. That hit home the most. Communication with Dipper, and how I embraced his journey, was all that was important. What amazing insights us humans can receive from totems.

The sadness never left my system, but seeing that symbolic figure gave me some relief. I didn't cry myself to sleep like usual. I actually fell deeply and comfortably in rest for the first time in weeks. And for the first time, I dreamt of my dear little Dipper! I couldn't pinpoint where we were at, but as soon as I walked in, I noticed him. The only thing was that he appeared to be in two different forms. In one, he looked exactly like I had remembered him. In the other, he was a bit younger and much healthier. Both versions were just as loving and courageous and gentle and distinctive to his personality. I couldn't believe that he was there with me. I could actually touch him, kiss him, and hug him. I didn't want to ever let go of him.

For Dipper, though, it was just like yesterday when we were playing in the hallway. He acted as if nothing had changed and we had never been separated. I wanted him to miss me and be excited to see me. He was enamored with my presence, but he carried on with zest and playfulness just like he always did at his favorite five o'clock hour. He didn't appear to feel an ounce of unhappiness. I couldn't comprehend what was going on. Then something came over me: HE WAS FREE!!!! I was watching him enjoy the grandest version of himself in his highest light. Talk about holding in a happy cry. I wanted to spend as much time with him as I could before the dream ended and the sun came up. I was consciously aware that I was in that state. Yet, it felt as real as ever. From that moment on, I understood that there was no difference in the space where we shared pure love and energy. It just seemed that way because I was focusing on his physicality.

Intuitively, the dream felt like it was coming to an end. Everything around us stopped and then both versions looked into my eyes and telepathically said to me, *"You have the choice how to remember me."* They both smiled and lit up with joy, and then my lids slowly lifted. My room was dark with a hint of blue light from his purifier. As I glanced towards the jackets hanging outside of the closet, a floating image appeared. I squinted as if to try and refocus, but it was Dipper. He was smiling the way he used to grin in his sleep, only with his eyes wide open. I quickly shut mine, then reopened them, and he was still there glistening with sparkles. I reached out my hands to softly rub the sides of his face, smiled back, and told him how much I loved him. I didn't blink again because I didn't want him to disappear. But before I knew it, the sun was shining through my blinds and he was gone.

I laid there for a while thinking about how beautiful he looked and how grateful I was that he came to visit. There was a calm, peaceful tone about the room. Something told me that he'd continue to show up from then on. For the whole month, I had sought to control the situation. I just wanted it all to have turned out differently. Then I realized that the key was releasing my attachment to his physical form and that one experience. Somehow, I allowed myself to receive the purest of love and, because so, his light found me. I could say that I unlocked a door to my heart and gained some strength to move ahead with a healthier mindset. But really, all I could do was surrender to the present moment and be in that space together. Here, or in the spirit world, we would be inseparable. Dipper didn't have to save me anymore. I was beginning to save myself.

I texted my parents and stepbrother to share the good news. I wasn't sure if my floaty boat had made it out of the ocean breakers and onto safer grounds, but I felt a hint of hope. The dogs and I went outside for our morning stretch, breath of fresh air, and the shimmering of the sun-risen sky. The scene and scent were moist just like I remembered in Los Angeles all those years. I was hoping to see my little green friend, but he was also gone. I guess he waited for the winds to settle before heading to his next destination and lucky recipient. He was the most phenomenal looking angel I had ever seen and was just as extraordinary in the messages he left me with. Something about his presence moved me... finally.

For the first time in a month, my entire day was peaceful and positive. I'd been a roller coaster of moods for four straight weeks. Yet, nothing seemed to shake my day. I even received an email in the afternoon stating that my mediation meeting had been pushed to December. That claim didn't mean anything to me anymore. I only decided to try and fight back as a means to give Dipper a better life. He was gone, so there was no reason to stay stuck to that energy. I let it go and trusted that whatever was meant to happen, would happen. Whatever wasn't, wouldn't.

I could tell that I was doing something right. Stuff that used to bother me wasn't bothering me anymore. Plus, my book was starting to evolve into something deeper. I could only write would I could through my pain, but it was beginning to take shape. Initially, it was therapy in helping me find the answers as to why my dog died. Then I thought about how it could benefit other people. Maybe others who had lost a pet could relate to my sadness. Maybe my experiences leading up to those final moments could help others deal with their own similar situations. I just wanted to help people get through their coping processes by traveling through mine. No matter how it would turn out, my book would always be a tribute to my little dog. Even if it was just for me... that would be all that mattered.

It became evident that I must've been releasing a ton of emotional toxins. My body was on fire as all aches had worsened. My joints hurt, my kneecaps burned, and my lower back was miserably stiff. My hair and nails were thinning, I wasn't sleeping, my cycles were out of whack, and I had severe toothaches. A lump developed, the top of my left foot seemed broken, and my breasts were tender and swollen. I'd been doing all the right things with binaural beats, silent meditations, mudras, emotional freedom tappings, writing, and acupuncture. I even forced myself to enjoy some laughter. In the nine hours my mom was at work, I would utilize all the self-healing techniques I could as a way of expressing and freeing up my cells. I hoped it would lessen the tension in my muscles, bones, organs, and meridians. Since the pain progressed to an almost unbearable state, I was either detoxing my system of polluted energy and built-up trauma... or so depressed, that I was creating illness and cancer.

I was praying that it meant I was putting myself back together. I had learned that things could be just as agonizing as when we're falling apart from the shifts my spine made after being exposed to toxic mold in the early 2000s. I had suffered from a multitude of symptoms for almost eight years, including rheumatoid arthritis, extreme bouts with vertigo, memory loss, and severe back pain by the final one. I took tons of tests with different practitioners. Aside from being entirely inflamed, it appeared that I had scoliosis and arthritis from injuries I sustained in the car accident from when I was a teen.

I was in complete shock because I hadn't ever experienced any pain in my back or body since. Thankfully, one of the alternative specialists advised me to move out of my apartment. Within 24-hours of relocating, things miraculously changed. In less than six months, I had no more cognition imbalances or aches anywhere, including my vertebrae. It took almost three years for me to fully recover and absorb nutrients. In that time, I struggled with similar highs and lows, both physically and mentally. One day, I'd be fine. The next, I was in crumbles. Then it would extend to one week. And the following, I was just as weak. Finally, I realized that I couldn't be going in two directions at once. I was either getting better or getting worse. That was the choice I had to make. The factor was shifting my perception.

I was sitting on the couch that evening thinking about what was ahead in the process, and if I could make it through. Then I remembered the wonderful Leaf Bug and his message to "just be patient." I missed Dipper so much. I missed us so much. I missed the synergy he brought to our entire Soular System. Although I had improved greatly in learning to embrace his new form, I couldn't help but revert. He had crossed the rainbow bridge and I was stuck in the mountains crossing the underpass at the end of a frontage road. I'd still think of dying on occasion. But it wasn't until I looked over to my sweet little Bodhi that I no longer let that thought consume me. With his big beautiful browns, he gazed up at my red face and bloodshot eyes and said, *"We're here too Mik. We need you too."*

Just like kids, we have other pets who are dependent on us. They need us... and love us... just as much.

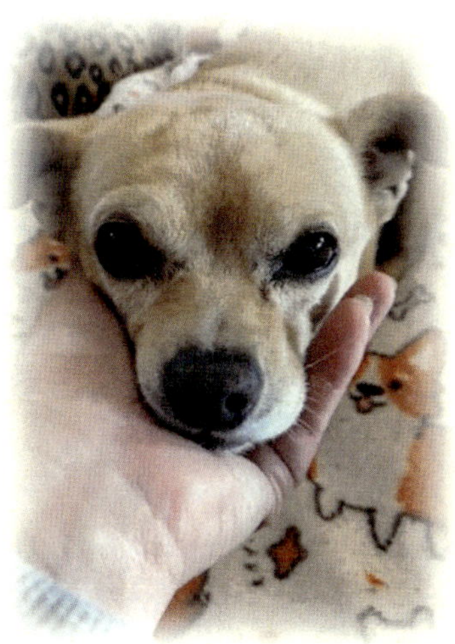

12
Awareness... Release... Lightness

It had been six weeks since Dipper died. How could time fly by so fast? How could life just go on without him? My days used to be so long after he left and now it was another sunrise in the middle of October. Mornings were some of our best times together. I wished that I could've just woken up out of my bad dream and it would've already been three o'clock in the afternoon. Yet, the world didn't stop for people's heartaches and losses. Highways kept going, stock markets crashed, baseball camps sprang up, and apps got developed. People got sober, renewed their vows, had babies, landed jobs, graduated, and rescued their soulmates. Since the 10th month usually meant new beginnings (10 → 1+0=1), then the cycle of life and death was inevitable. I still had my sweet Bodhi and Lola. And just like always, something else would come along to take my attention in a different direction.

I had contacted a grief counselor a couple weeks earlier based on the suggestion from one of my acupuncturists. Never had I gone to a psychologist or any other type of emotional therapist. For one, I couldn't afford it. Secondly, I always soldiered on with healthy food, exercise, self-help tools, and natural, alternative therapeutics. I made the best of what I could with what I had. But I was a mess.

Since my dad died, my life seemed to be continually sinking. The only areas that worked for me were writing motivational stories and when I was helping to uplift others. Whether through energy work, fitness training, or recently saving animals, I felt successful. Those moments allowed me to come up for air and gain back enough enthusiasm to keep paddling. Then Dipper stepped into the picture and the good parts of the story became a consistent focus. That was because he wasn't just a moment. He was momentous. The problem was that I hadn't fully recovered from my past disaster, and then got hit with his death. Talk about a snowball of life storms back to visit.

I didn't know how the counselor understood a thing I said in that first phone consultation. I couldn't get more than three sentences out before hyperventilating and exploding into tears. Somehow, I made it to my third online session. We had spent each appointment going through a lengthy questionnaire. The topics were simple and appeared to have nothing to do with my current situation. She asked about my interests, work experience, goals, social abilities, relationships, and friendships. Then we got into my take on team-work, lineage, childhood happenings, and personal viewpoints. As we went through each inquiry, I found myself discovering things about myself that I hadn't remembered. I'm sure she expected short answers. But aspects of specific outcomes, and the reasons behind them, were coming back to me. That was probably why we were on session #3 and had only gotten halfway through the worksheet.

Then, something began to make sense. I had obviously pushed a lifetime of subconscious thoughts and hidden trauma into my system, and stored them somewhere in my organs. I could say that my brain was the culprit in removing those ordeals from my mind so that other areas of my body could function. But I repeatedly had issues with my liver, spleen, large intestine, pericardium, pancreas, digestion, and even cholesterol. I always related it to the depression that I developed from losing my dad and never picking up that last phone call. It was almost always the target assessed through acupuncture.

But like a light bulb going off, I realized that it was about more than just that one experience. It was about all the deaths and losses, in every form, that I had experienced. It was about people who passed, jobs I didn't get, credit and respect I didn't receive, loss of income, and residences I had to move out of. It also related to the times when my health went bad, I missed opportunities, my self-esteem and independence declined, and all the dogs that were removed from my life. It was an accumulation of emotions stuck in one big coping process. How could my *Qi* not be depleted? Every pattern of pain and struggle that I had experienced was connected. Like most of us, I thought I did my best to get better after each misfortune. But I never made it out of the first six islands of healing. For me to get to a place of peace, I'd have to release and accept... and find forgiveness.

I had to begin by forgiving myself for thinking that I killed my own dog. I gave him drugs that I knew would kill him, but he could've also died from withholding them. I would've felt just as awful and blamed myself just as much. The medication may have caused him the tormenting ending, but he could've also had just as tragic of a closing from not taking them. I only wanted to save my dog. Everything I had done was to harmonize every single part of his beingness. He was every part of mine. So, why would I think that any decision I made at any other time would contradict what my intent was all along?

I hated that he died, how he died, why he died, and when he died. But he died. Just like humans, I had always believed that we went when we did regardless of how the illusion presented itself. I had never been through something that traumatic with someone I loved so much, so I guess I forgot. I had to remember what I always believed about death, and let go of the hazardous emotions attached to that one last act and decision. I had to release myself of the horrendous guilt and choose to see, accept, and embrace the experience in a softer sense. That way it wouldn't turn into another form of repressed damage lining my insides with plaque.

It took me almost two decades to be okay with not picking up the last call from my dad. I wasn't going to fully be able to let myself off the hook in two months for what I did to Dipper. Yet, I knew where I had to take my soul. I knew what lay ahead and the power I had in shifting a pattern that kept me feeling like I was always suffering. Maybe not in the way I would've chosen but, again, I was offered another opportunity to make things right. Like with my dogs from when I was a kid, I wasn't going to mess it up again. I had lots of work ahead of me in breaking down years' worth of subconscious blocks in order to finally reach a place of true peace and happiness. If anything, I just wanted to get back into a balanced state well enough with myself, that the next time everything seemingly fell apart... I wouldn't.

For the first time in months, maybe even years, I felt like I got an answer. I was still stuck in many ways, but I finally got a solid answer. Forgiving myself for my most recent experience was only the beginning. I had to go back in time to address other situations that changed the direction of a path I had been attached to. I never felt like there was any benefit in going backwards or revisiting pasts for any reasons other than to reminisce on amazing memories. Yet, my current self had to return back to my previous self for a timeline of brief moments... in order to free my present self of the in between areas of pain and struggle. I had to find a way to see the middle as more pleasant. To do that, I'd have to find a way back to my heart.

I didn't know if I had one more dinghy to help get me through the last three islands, but something told me I wouldn't need them. I had survived the darkest corners of grief up to that point and was entering new doors of unfamiliar territory. I was ready to fly again. I knew release and acceptance would be challenging. Therefore, I wanted to make sure I'd at least get streaming animal rescue videos, coconut pancakes, and an aromatherapy massage. Peaceful Island was on my horizon. I just had to choose which mindset I'd take to get me there.

The most soothing luggage I could've packed included the book I had begun writing and four poster-sized boards filled with Dipper's pictures. I didn't want to take him away from the space of pure love and energy he was in, so I began putting together photo collages on wall-sized cardboards. His essence was always with me, but I didn't want him to become a faint memory. As I began scrolling through the thousands of pictures and videos I had of him, I was brought back to all the better times with him. What a lightness it gave to my heart. He was the best work of art I ever created. I used to laugh at people who had thousands of pictures of their newborns on their phones. How I was eating my words. I had enough images to make 50 boards, but I kept it to four and in chronological order. They were blue and added so much life to my room; just as if he was there in person.

It was a bit weird how some of the photos of him sleeping were almost identical to when he was dormant the night he died. I never noticed the few times he had the same hollow depth in his eyes, because he was usually smiling. He was such a darling spectacle to watch when he got lost in rest. There was nothing beautiful about life leaving his body. But after I put his tongue back in his mouth, closed his jaw, and softly shut his lids, the gentleness of the air returned as he laid there motionless. Just like when in breath, it was as if his calm intuition knew I was right next to him making sure nothing happened.

After making those boards, I stayed staring at his charming little face. There wouldn't be anything I could do to make me miss him less. But those pics helped. Although the guilt of getting better still eroded my insides, I knew I was on my way to reaching some kind of light. I had to. He taught me how to. When I first got Dipper, he had nothing left going for him. Yet, he still chose to fully live. Look how beautiful things ended up with him. And that was after someone gave up on him. There was no way I could let him down and give up on myself.

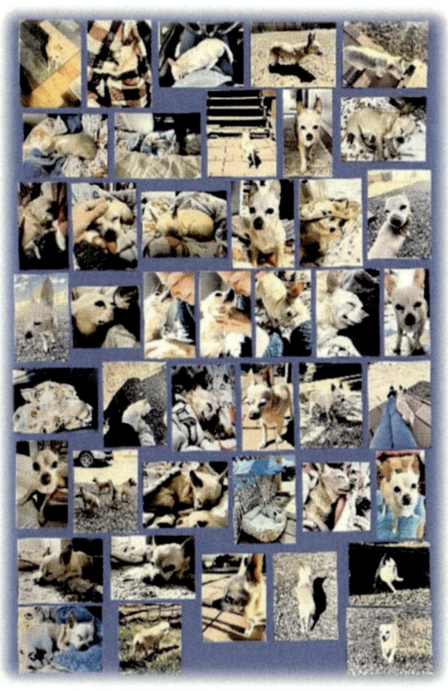

My beeswax candles were burning out, so I turned off the lamp and let them finish off the night for us. Bodhi cuddled up next to my pillow while Lola snuck into the covers. I was already a few minutes into crying myself to sleep when he looked up at me to say, *"Why are you so sad? You still have us."* I took a moment and a breath. How lucky did I get with that little guy? He never left my side. I felt pathetic that I wasn't at a place where I could give him the time like I gave to Dipper. I still kissed his sweet face a million times a day and let him know that he was always my number one. I just had to work on myself so that I could get there again and give him just as much love.

In the middle of the night, I woke up to him moving around nervously. He usually slept straight into the morning. But when he whined, I knew it was his way of letting me know he had to poop. I wasn't surprised because he ate part of my homemade bean and cheese red chili burrito earlier. We walked outside and it was a bit chilly. The midnight sky was dark blue and the stars were brilliant. For some reason, Bodhi wouldn't go down the stairs to take his shit in his regular spot. He just stood there looking back at me like, *"Hurry up."* The dude had woken me up in a panic so that he could go outside to handle business, and now he was stalling for whatever the reason.

He was a baby sometimes. And like a little kid, he just needed me to hold his paw. I walked over to him and we went down the steps together. And what do you know? The Little Dipper was out! That constellation used to shine down on us every single night when Dip was alive. It had been the first time those stars showed up in over six weeks. They were glowing so intense that the frigid air didn't bother me. I just wanted to sleep outside so that I could be right next to him.

While I was stuck in my trance, my other dogs were done being outside and already scratching on the screen door. I said goodbye to my little boy and told him how much I loved and missed him. We got back into bed and, surprisingly, fell asleep instantly. Then, just as quickly, life turned into another dream. I was back outside looking for the Little Dipper up in the same midnight sky. Instead of the 7-point configuration looking like a spatula, it formed the words, "I Love You." Right below, there was another set of stars in the shape of Dipper's face. He was smiling. Just like my other dream, he came to show me how I could remember him. There wouldn't be anything better about my life without having him in the flesh, but I would be better than I was yesterday because of him. The signs, stars, messages, totems, and dreams were slowly bringing me back to a place of peace.

By that time, we were a few days from completing the month and football was the highlight of our family unit. My parents had always loved sporting events and Sundays were our days to make our bets, cook fabulous meals, spoil the dogs with yummy treats, and share an abundance of great energy. They were also days that took my mind away, so I appreciated them and my family more than ever.

My stepbrother would make the hour and a half trip from the metro city to spend every Sunday with us. We were only three years apart and you would've thought we grew up around the same groups of people. Yet, that wasn't the case at all. We had a cool familiarity with one another, but I never really got to know his mind in extent. I had been in Los Angeles the entire time and only saw him on the holidays like everyone else. My dad did though. He and my father shared an amazing friendship. I knew they'd have wisdom talks on a whole other level on days that they'd play chess. They discussed the mechanics and psychology of life, but also shared their views and opinions regarding relationships and women.

My dad was an unbelievably charismatic dude with a giant heart. He could make friends with the walls. He was also extremely intelligent, loved fishing, the outdoors, and was an outstanding musician. He reeked of art, knowledge, youthfulness, and out-of-the-box thinking. It was no wonder that they'd have such a close bond. It was somewhat father-like, but my dad wanted to make sure not to cross any boundaries between him and his own dad. My dad was best friends with my mom and stepdad, and had all the respect in the world for both of them. He was well aware that my stepbrother and my stepfather had their own connective similarities and differences. It was awesome that all four of them could enjoy friendships with each other for their own reasons.

Since living back home with my parents, him and I had also developed an incredible friendship. I really enjoyed the exchanges we would have every game day. He was also one of the only persons I kept in contact with after losing Dipper. He'd always send meaningful texts offering love and support. I hadn't trusted the timing of anything those days. As I continued improving mentally, I began putting it together that even he came into my life accordingly.

Unfortunately, he was the one that found my dad's body. My dad and stepdad were preparing to drive to Denver that following morning for a quick trip. But after not hearing from him, my stepdad knew something was wrong. He called my mom at work and they both decided to ask my stepbrother if he'd stop by to check on him. He was at the office, and wasn't able to get to my dad's until about 3pm.

He knew something wasn't right because my dad's car was out front with the house doors still locked. He walked around to see if he noticed anything unusual. Then he headed to the back of the trailer to try and peek in through the tiny window. That's when he saw my dad laying on the bathroom floor. It appeared that he'd been there for quite some time. He immediately drove to a nearby phone and called the cops and our parents. Since he found my dad, he was questioned for hours. By the time all three of them were released to go home, it was close to midnight. I had no idea how that process affected any of them. I was busy packing and making plane flights to get home the next morning.

My stepbrother told me that my dad and him would always speak about "the other side." They both agreed that there was some type of afterlife, but they weren't sure how communication could be confirmed. Other people always had their own stories and experiences, but how many of those inquiries were shams? Was there a way to prove it to each other? They came up with a pact that whoever left first would have to come back in some way and give a sign that the other side existed. After my stepbrother returned to his apartment that night, the first thing he wanted to do was take a shower and rinse off the energy of death. Then he put on his jammies and jumped into bed. As exhausted as he was, he struggled to fall asleep. His best buddy had just died and he couldn't get the images out of his mind. Finally, he dozed off around 1:30am.

He was suddenly awakened by a loud noise. He thought someone had broken into his apartment. The bedroom was pitch black, so he didn't know if anybody was in his room or not. He was frozen with fear. After waiting a few minutes, he didn't hear any more sounds. He took a few deep breaths and was able to sit up. Then he reached over to turn on the light. That's when he saw that one of the shelves on his bookcase had broken, and all of the books were scattered everywhere. Oddly enough, the book that landed closest to his feet was about how to succeed with women. Instantly, he was relieved that someone hadn't broken in after all. He was also stunned. Why would that particular book be the one that stood out? Was it the sign he and my dad spoke about? Or, was it just a coincidence?

He headed for the bathroom to splash some water on his face. When he looked in the mirror, he was completely pale. He had only turned on the switch for the regular light, but decided to turn on the heat lamp in hopes of getting some color back. The second he flipped on the switch, the bulb exploded and glass shattered all over the floor. There he was staring at himself, petrified, thinking, "What just happened?" That's when he became convinced that my dad showed up to give him a sign. He didn't expect it to pop up that soon. My dad had just died. Wasn't it supposed to take a few days for his spaceship to burst through the atmosphere? It hadn't even been twenty-four hours and he was back. It was like he had never left.

The next afternoon, my stepbrother decided to hit the gym. He felt like it was the only way to grasp any sense of normalcy. He was still in shock, and couldn't believe that my dad was gone. After his workout, he went straight back to his apartment. As he began taking things out of his bag, he realized that his wallet was gone. He couldn't find it anywhere. So, he drove back to the fitness center to see if anyone had turned it in. Surprisingly, someone had. Nothing was missing. His driver's license, credit cards, and money were still intact. He asked if the person left a name? Maybe he could repay him or her for their kindness. The employee told him that it was a guy named Ernest. That was my dad's name. He said right there that he knew. That was the third sign they had talked about and concrete proof that my dad made good on his promise. He said that it was actually a gift of faith and hope, and left him with a powerful thing to believe in.

It would be no accident that my stepbrother found him. My dad wouldn't have wanted it any other way. That was the kind of bond they had in life and in death. Not only was I a walking part of my dad, but so was he. My mom and stepdad were as well. That was the kind of impact my dad had on us and the legacy he left us with. I looked forward to hearing more about my stepbrother's insights to the spirit world and sharing stories of similar phenomena from Dipper. Those like-minded talks were good for my soul. Not many people had ever understood me, my beliefs, or my outlooks on life. I was quickly finding out that he would be one of the few that actually got me.

The few others that I was having conversations with to that magnitude were my friend Alana, my acupuncturists, and my grief counselor. They were all compassionate and understanding of the grieving process. They also saw eye-to-eye on spirituality. I was beyond grateful to have them in my corner supporting me. Yet, I knew it would be the last of my healing sessions. I could've said that I didn't want to borrow any more money from my mom to pay for them, but I knew by the third meeting that I wouldn't be going any further. In that short amount of time, I was able to connect with what I needed.

In no way was I dissatisfied with any part of her program. I had never received such beneficial information about myself through a simple questionnaire. It took five meetings to complete the worksheet that she designed to help strategize a plan for me. What she didn't realize, was that those questions were better than any therapy she could've given me. They revealed parts of my past that I hadn't fully cleared and closed. Maybe I didn't think of them as being as important. Or maybe, I just moved on and made the best of them. I was able to begin seeing the reasons and backstories to all of them, and why they led to how I responded to loss and death up to that point in my life. I was about to face myself even more and begin revisiting times where I went against my gut, and made decisions, that altered my path and the paths of others I loved.

Going back in time wasn't going to be easy by any means. I was still working through a grueling process of forgiving myself for cutting off Dip's electricity. My heart was tender. What I had to remember was that I never intended for any of my choices to take a turn for the worse; not with him, or with anything in my life. I had mentioned earlier in the book that, ***"We get where we get when we do. Where we grow is in the middle."*** The beginning and ending of anything are inevitable, especially for a pet. For me to find solace in any of my unfavorable past outcomes, I had to reconnect with everything beautiful in between. That meant having to release myself from thinking I needed the whys of everything on the outside.

I knew I had a number of decisions to begin working through, but a handful stood out. Charly and Tippet were two of the most important. I had spent three amazing years with those precious dogs.

Day in and day out, I reassured them that I would never leave them. Yet, I did. And I didn't do what it took to keep them. I hated that we were forced to part ways and I hated even more that they were alive, without me, and living with someone who didn't deserve them. They taught me how powerful love was by how much somebody would sacrifice for it. That somebody being me, would have done anything for them. Never had I felt a love that powerful about anyone other than my parents and best friend. On the other hand, they taught me that there was nothing, or no one, you could love so deeply that it would take jeopardizing yourself. Because of them, I would never allow anyone to misuse me again. That was a promise I would keep.

They were the link that reconnected me with my childhood love for animals and, as a result, I went on to adopt Bodhi, Lola, and Dipper. I was able to extend the quality of life for three more dogs because they showed me how to do it. I would've liked for it to have gone a different way, but thank goodness my love influenced others to love them even more. That was all I could've wished for... was that they were well-taken care of. I had to release myself from the remorse and sadness I carried for breaking my word to them. I had to free myself of the guilt that ate me up for not fighting to keep them. I regretted so many things that, if I had done differently, they'd still be with me. All three of us ended up where we did. I just had to remember what we shared in the middle.

When it came to my past relation entanglement, there wasn't anything substantial within the starting and ending points except for Char and Tip, and the dearness I shared with his father. I still had to go back and forgive myself for getting involved in the first place. I had no idea what I was committing to, but I knew from the onset that it didn't feel right. I also knew not to give up my dreams or compromise any part of me. Yet, I did. Because so, I lost everything, including myself, temporarily. The regret and disappointment were consuming my world. I couldn't allow the shame and embarrassment of allowing someone to control and compress me... to continue weighing heavily on my soul. I took a chance and it didn't work out. I had to finally let go of my attachment to that mega mistake, and release myself from giving it any more credit of where I was currently at.

Since I had gotten my mother involved in property loans and investment transactions, I also had a good amount of guilt and blame lodged deep in my gut. She even put her professional reputation on the line to help us out even more, by helping to increase my ex's gross income. She ended up getting sued in the process. She was a grown woman who made her own choices, but she was still my mom. I felt terrible. All she had ever done in her life was to help better mine. I was sorry that I had brought her into my partnership. Yet, I had to let go of feeling responsible for how it turned out. I had no idea I was gonna get duped, much less her. We both did our best in hopes of my relationship being successful. There was nothing more I could feel at fault for. I still wanted her to take legal action due to the strength of her case. But she had a gift of not hanging on to shit. She also believed in karma and the cyclic nature of cause and effect. Therefore, there were plenty of others to share our energy and court fees with.

When it came to my tv and film career, the release process brought me back to another load of letdowns. I was honored and humble for the shows I booked, getting called in by amazing casting directors, and being repped by a few fantastic agents. That's why I went out there. But after years of paying dues, chasing prosperity, and dealing with overwhelming competition and rejection, I wasn't connecting with spiritual substance. And because so, I always felt stuck; both in mind and in body. I questioned why I stayed glued to that scene for so long since my gut would constantly tell me to do something else. Plus, the drive, determination, and hope that kept me attached in the beginning were fading. I also settled my beingness immensely by the personal choices I made in allowing others to devalue me.

I began thinking that maybe I didn't really love that occupation, but just needed to feel important like when I was a kid. The problem was that I had already put all my eggs in one basket, stayed planted, and misspent so many new moons by never wavering in trying to get on the big screen. I was going to do what it took as long as it didn't undermine who I was, what I believed in, my safety, and my mental health. All that did was keep me from getting noticed. I was filled with a plethora of talents. Yet, I didn't open myself up to healthier opportunities, including working with animals.

I had to take back my power and belief in who I was, and choose a more optimistic perception of how well I did. I went out to one of the largest cities in the world and explored a goal that many people didn't have the balls to do. I was good enough to be hired for national projects, so I was exactly what they wanted. I taught myself how to write screenplays and television sitcoms, I wrote and published a few books, and I also started fitness training and energy guidance work. Having the guts to go out there all alone, and continue to persist no matter the odds, were no joke. I didn't sell out, and didn't waste anything by keeping my focus on one thing. Just because I didn't make it how I would've liked to then, didn't mean the end of me. Those were prime years of absorption. I was given loads of tools to ripen and reinvent myself in so many ways. And because so, I was able to help a ton of people feel better about themselves. I had to remember the positive impact I had on that single microcosmic period in time.

As for my dad, mom, and stepdad, they never understood what I saw in Hollywood. Yet, that didn't stop them from standing by me and my aspirations regardless of how far-fetched they were. My mom spent her savings and tax returns to help keep me there, not to mention the pure emotional support. How blessed was I to have her? I felt bad for not being as gentle with her, and when I pushed her to be someone that she wasn't. It was time to unleash needing to understand her formulas, and simply treasure the time I had with her.

Lastly, I had my beloved Rudy. How could I abandon him and leave him tied to a tree? How could I take him for granted and not make him my priority? I had to admit that I was never able to get those sad visuals out of my mind. He was so innocent and even more confused that his human left him. I wish I would've acted differently, but I didn't. I had to finally be okay with myself for how it turned out. Because my dad gave him away, he connected with someone who was able to make his life wonderful in every way. That went for Fritz and Peaches as well. I had aways harbored sorrow for being so irresponsible. I had to cut those ties and let that heaviness go. There were too many other great memories with them to think back on. Because of my actions, they landed in a home with people who were able to be more present with them. It turned into a win for everyone.

I knew I had more rubble in my system. But for the moment, I was done dissecting myself for going against my gut and making turns that became detours. I could've done more, better, and stood up for myself on so many levels, but I couldn't change any of it. All I could do was release it, embrace it, and be alright with me. No matter where those decisions relocated me, or others, I had to let go of giving them power. It was my choice to see certain parts of my past with a brighter lens, so that my present and future wouldn't suffer.

I was starting to feel like I could breathe again. The tightness in my diaphragm was loosening. I knew I was making strides, and that was because my focus was on healing from what I did, not what others did. Some people have been able to forgive all involved, but I wasn't there yet. I didn't feel that action to be my responsibility. I certainly didn't feel like it would bring me peace. It was more important to work on breaking the chains hovering over my own soul from my own decisions. No matter how big or small the loss or mishap, I had to find a way to come to grips with the aftermath. It would be nice if those that hurt us were genuinely sorry and could somehow make up for it. But that's a foolish expectation. People would pay their karmic dues in this lifetime or the next. And that weight would be theirs to carry, not mine. I wouldn't forgive them for what they did, but I'd let go of holding them accountable for the direction my path took from it.

In Dipper's case, I couldn't fault anyone for trying to do their best. Maybe his previous human gave him up in hopes that he'd have a better life and home. Maybe the shelter did what they did thinking he'd become more adoptable. Even though the vet at the clinic overdosed him with meds, and then had me overdose him, she was trying to save him. She told me she wasn't familiar with homeopathic healing. Clearly, she was taught to administer drugs as a way of treatment. But I had to admit that she was always extra kind to him. I was especially appreciative when that lump had to be removed from the back of his thigh and she chose not to put him under anesthesia. There wasn't a vet in town that would've done that. Yet, she did, and I would forever be grateful for her gentleness. She sent me a condolence card after he died stating how sad the entire office was of his passing. I was pissed, so it didn't register that they hurt too.

Then there were all those times when my stepdad would tell me to wait until Dipper stopped eating and started going downhill. I couldn't stand being around that nauseating energy. But as I looked back, it was just his way of alerting me of the harsh reality that he had experienced with his own pets. He was protecting me from feeling as awful as I felt. I was sorry that I saw his compassion so differently. Release and acceptance were such hard pills to swallow, but shedding off that heavy weight had become liberating. It was interesting how so many things didn't make sense. Then, they started making sense.

I began to remember that Dipper got sick too. He had "off" days and a few days that I thought might be his last days. Most days, he was peppy, robust, and filled with and abundance of joy. A few of the others, he was unstable and fragile. I guess I got caught up in the miracles he was accomplishing on almost all days.

Then there were the signs that kept coming as his transformation drew closer. Yet, I still thought I could have him longer. From the furry black caterpillar, to the *Día de Los Muertos* cushion, to the emotional Monday, I was being sent messages to prepare. Then, there was the mosquito planted on his nose to show me that he was too weak to keep them from sucking the life out of him. There were all the times he continued to gravitate to the light, even so much as falling through the stairs from trying to reach the sun. He got so ill the day before his birthday, that his little body laid limp on the rug with his tongue sticking out, his eyes half-shut, and his lungs struggling to pump air. He looked so similar after he died, as if readying me for that image.

He almost turned his head back a few days before his last and had never done that before. It was like he wanted to tell me something, but realized that he couldn't alter his natural course of time. On the day before he left, he took his usual walk to the front door, but hesitated from stepping onto the deck. He stood there for a few minutes before tears began to flood his eyes. He looked so sad and so beautiful at the same time. It was as if he was struggling with something inside. Then he closed his lids and became a vision of a pure white angel. A little later that afternoon, I thought it was cute that he began sitting down to eat his food. I had no idea that he was losing the strength of his kidneys and the lower portion of his spine.

A couple weeks before he died, I'd been watching a Netflix show called, *Surviving Death*. The series surrounded people that were having difficulties coping with the loss of their loved ones. Each episode focused on stages of the experience. Some went into detail about the initial shock people got hit with. Others included various emotions people delt with. I mostly felt that those shows were an accumulation of messages explaining to us that there was actually another side we could communicate with.

Many of the people on those episodes were overcome with sadness. Some had made it through a few of the first islands and had reached another level to their healing. Others couldn't get out of the first few and were painfully stuck. I remembered having a pit in my stomach as to why I was watching that series, and why I was so interested. After Dipper passed, it became clear. I'd soon be in the same position as those heartbroken family members just praying for him to send me a sign that he was with me.

He had just reached his nineteenth year of enlightenment. He had progressed so quickly, and seemed to have beaten all the odds, that I thought I could have him forever. I lost track of the reason I brought him into our hearts and our home in the first place: I didn't want him to die in a shelter by himself. His time was coming sooner than I wanted to believe... and forever for us ended up being 5 ½ months.

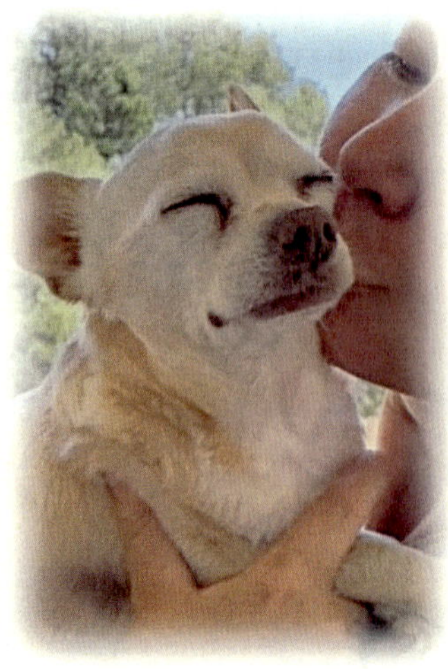

13
Gratitude:
The Gateway to Pure Love and Energy

Just like March had become April, then May, June, July, and August when Dipper was alive, September became November just as fast. We had entered the 11th month and the colors were shifting. The leaves had fallen and the notorious wind found its way back to our address. How I despised that wind and all it blew in. I also dreaded the freezing cold temperatures. That piercing air was already seeping in through the window sills. Nothing had been the same since Dip died, but I was increasingly making progress each day. The more emotional weight I continued to release through forgiveness and acceptance, the more subconscious blocks I broke down and eliminated. It was like shedding layers of skin that had thickened since I was a kid.

I was beginning to remember the great things I had gone through, and the great decisions I made, over what I could've done differently. The sad parts to my story were turning into triumphs. It had only been a little over two months since losing my little boy and I was laughing, socializing a bit through texts, and enjoying things I had forgotten to enjoy. I had a long way to go in my recovery, but at least I was going. As an actress all those years in Hollywood, I always used to hear that life imitated art. If I could've summed up the point I was currently at, I'd have to recite the lyrics from one of my favorite songs, *November Rain*, by Guns N' Roses. They were the dialogue to my next scene:

"And when your fears subside
And shadows still remain,
I know that you can love me when there's no one left to blame.
So never mind the darkness, we still can find a way
Cuz nothin' lasts forever, even cold November rain."

There was no doubt that it had been a continuous storm. Yet, for the first time, in a long time, the waves had calmed. We had entered a new cycle of the moon phase and it just happened to land on month eleven. I had always associated the mystical number of "11" with angels. It first began visiting me in repeating patterns *(1111)* the year my dad transitioned. I hadn't ever seen them so predominantly or frequently, so I knew they had something to tell me.

I began studying the recurring numbers that kept showing up so that I could see what the deeper meaning and purpose were to their visits. Almost everything I ran across listed "11" as a master number, which resonated at an extremely high vibration. I knew the number "1" represented new beginnings, change, initiatives, and leadership. So, doubling the double of it had to be pretty powerful. I had just turned 26 years of age, and was going through the most difficult time of my life. I began to view those numbers as a form of protection and guidance from the spirit world. In a sense, they acted as a security cushion from my guardian winged fairies. Or, it was just my dad coming back as a ghost to help me get through losing him.

Those numbers symbolized the depth of soulness. They represented pure reflection – connection – and oneness to me. I learned that the numeric messages came to offer me a spiritual awakening, presence, and wholeness. They were also the first of my rebirths, and the beginning of connecting the physical plane with my internal consciousness. Even though I'd see them every so often throughout different phases in my life, it would be no wonder that they'd come back just as prevalent right after Dipper died. Even better... he began to show up just as often!

I'd see the numbers everywhere. They were on clocks, my cell phone, my laptop, and minutes and seconds left on the quarters of football games. They'd be on the oven timers, my step counter, the change left over, and the time and date of my next acupuncture appointment. Then, I began to notice that channels were changed on the television set in my bedroom. I was the only one who used that tv. One night I even saw a dogfood commercial with a puppy who looked exactly like Dipper at a younger age. He was wearing a similar green hoodie like the one we dressed him in after his first bath. He'd pop up in my acupuncture sessions and blow cold air in my left ear. He'd shake the bed, and also steam himself into the texture of my elephant painting that hung on the wall behind my headboard. I'd catch Bodhi staring at that piece for minutes at a time. Always, he would be smiling.

I had decided to go through with a laser eye procedure two weeks after Dipper died. I know, who does that right? But the appointment had been made in July and the doctor was booked up for months. My vision began getting blurry when I was involved in my relationship. Since my adrenal glands were also currently shot, I related both to the stress I was going through. After Dip turned into stardust, I lost interest. I didn't feel like I was in any kind of condition to be having surgery, even if it was only a touch up. But for some reason, I still went through with it and the experience turned out to be hilarious.

The team gave me a few relaxing pills to loosen me up before the two-minute procedure, so I already felt drunk by the time I sat in the chair. Afterwards, they sent me home with a powerfully prescribed sedative to keep me from opening my eyes. I wasn't too keen on taking meds, but that was how my cornea would heal. The reason I didn't speak about it before was because I passed out for two full days and didn't have any recollection of anything. I decided to mention it now because as Dipper began visiting, so did flashes of light. Most of the time, they'd whiz right by me. I'd look around thinking I was going crazy. But then those flashes would whiz by again and again. I didn't know if it was because I tampered with my right lens, or if Dip was showing off in his new form.

I didn't think it had anything to do with the laser because he'd also appear as white and blue orbs. The white ones would swing from wall to wall in my bedroom at different times of the day regardless of the weather outside. We lived in the middle of nowhere, so there wasn't a lot of traffic. That also meant that there wasn't much movement to catch a glare in between the blinds. Birds didn't hang out on our side of the property either because we didn't have the luxurious feeding oasis that my stepdad had for them on his side. That guy was so good with animals and nature that every creature from all walks of life couldn't wait for a spot to open up so that they could move in.

The bright blue orbs began showing up on the ceiling when I started writing in the living room. They looked like lymphocytes, and were so mesmerizing because they were blue. That's how I knew it was Dip. They'd stay dormant just waiting for me to pay attention. Once I'd focus my eyes on them for more than a few seconds, they would divide. It was like the more I gave them energy, the more they came alive and spread out. I even took videos from my cell phone because I knew nobody was going to believe me. When they watched the phenomena, they were in awe.

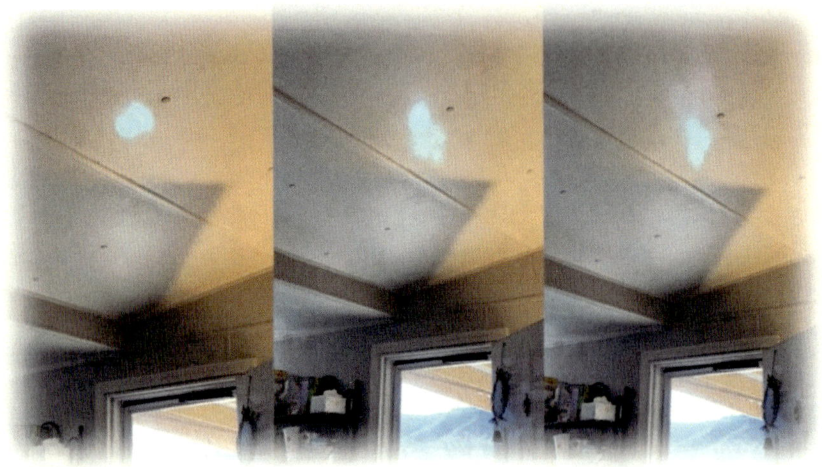

What really blew my mind was the night Dip showed up in real life. Both dogs slept in bed with me, but Lola was on her own schedule and moods. She'd been spending the evenings with my mom for a week, and stayed with her in the bed a few nights. She became a sweet little thing, but still had a hot temper. As much as she soaked up the spoiling from my mom, she'd switch faces and the exorcist would come out. Before I knew it, she'd be scratching at my door to come in after I had already fallen deep into my sleep realm. I really needed to get my rest since I was mentally drained. So, my mom started putting up the doggy gate to keep her from bothering me.

One night, I was ready to pass out early and actually put the gate up myself. Lola didn't notice because she was burrowed underneath my mom's blanket while they were watching tv on the couch. In the middle of the night, I woke up to both Bodhi and Lola sleeping against my right leg. I remembered thinking, how in the world didn't I hear my mom come in and put Lola in bed with me? She deserved an award for that. Just like that hour every night, neither her or Bodhi moved. They were deep in their own sleep zones. I laid there for about ten minutes with my hands on both of them thinking how attached they were to me, as I was to them. We sure were lucky to have each other. Then I fell asleep thinking about Dip.

By the time morning came, I was awakened by Lola barking at the dogs outside. Again, I thought to myself, how in the world did my mom come into my room and take that girl out without me hearing her? I had ears like an owl. I could catch what my stepdad was saying on the phone fifty yards away. I must've really been tired. When I got out of bed and opened my door to tell Lola to shut the "F" up, the gate was still up. I asked my mom if she placed it there that morning, and she hadn't. Lola slept with her all night. She let her outside once the sun came up. I realized right then that I wasn't dreaming. Lola had never come back into my room. It was Dipper.

I had always heard that your loved ones didn't come back to communicate with you until you were ready. My dad had appeared in a dream the week I returned to LA. He was waiting for me in a parking lot, so we both hopped into my red Toyota truck. Before anything, I asked him if he knew he was going to die? He nodded, "Yes," and then everything went straight to a black screen. Instantly, I woke up. After that, he only showed up periodically. So, I didn't quite know what "ready" meant. But I was well aware that I had opened a door which would allow me to receive Dipper fully. I knew he'd also go on and only come to me periodically. Until then, I was going to savor every single moment he made his entrance.

It was the 11th and I had forgotten that it was Veteran's Day. I had to cancel my acupuncture appointment because we usually spent it going to the National Cemetery to visit, and pay tribute, to all those loved ones that my stepdad lost. I knew I'd get a chance to see my ex's father as well. The last time I got to be with him was at his funeral, and we all know how that went. What I didn't realize was that death was upon us once again.

My stepdad called early and we thought maybe it was because he wanted to start the day sooner. Yet, he sounded somber. He told us that he was going to put Selena down. I couldn't believe what I was hearing. I knew that she had unexpectedly begun having some type of spasms a few days earlier. She was walking through the yard when she suddenly fell and began seizing. She had never done that before. That previous afternoon, I was sitting out on his porch while he was fixing the gate. She fell over right in front of me. She began panting and trying to reach out her arms, but they just went stiff. She was so helpless. It brought back the night Dipper took his last stretch.

I desperately wanted him to try other options to see if we could keep her alive. I didn't feel it was her time. But she wasn't my dog, and his mind was made up. He had been through the process many times before and didn't want her to suffer. She was such a beautiful, gentle soul. I hated that we were going to have to part ways with her.

I hadn't stepped foot anywhere near that clinic since Dipper died, but I had to show up for her. I had to admit that it helped that the doctor had retired, but I still felt an eeriness walking through those doors. Selena was so scared. She had no idea that she was about to exit our family earth. When we got settled in, they placed an IV in her leg and, within minutes, her energy and spirit seemed to elevate. She looked peppy and youthful, just like we were used to seeing her. It reminded me of how radiant Dipper looked in that same office on his last day. I had heard that people and pets would sometimes get a burst of unexplained energy before departing; making it even more difficult to let them go. I had just gone through it myself, so I knew.

The new doctor walked in and she seemed much softer. We picked up Selena and put her on the table. That's when her nervousness sunk in. The solution was inserted into the catheter and we spent the next minute cupping her sweet face, and telling her what a good girl she was and how much we loved her. Then she slowly fell asleep. It wasn't peaceful by any means. But as tears overflowed our face masks, I was grateful that she didn't suffer a painful exit. I had never seen a dog euthanized before and transition out of their body in that way. It made me think that maybe it would've been better to have done that with Dipper. I just didn't know how his final moments would unravel.

For a moment, guilt tried to creep back in for being so selfish. Because really, I forced him to stick around. Every time he tried to leave, I would do everything to keep him there with me. I knew that he stayed as long as he could just to make me happy. His 19th birthday was more important to me than it was to him. Therefore, I had one more thing I had to forgive myself for... and that would be for trying so hard to keep him with me when he kept showing us that he was ready to go. I couldn't beat myself up anymore for taking the path I did. I had to be okay with the fact that I thought I was doing the right thing and with the intentions only to help him; not to hurt him.

It was November 11th (11/11) and those numbers continued to be connective. For some reason, Dipper had issues with Selena. Not always. But every so often, he'd show his manliness by trying to bark and throttle himself towards her. We couldn't figure out if she reminded him of an ex-girlfriend or if it was his way of flirting. She never minded though. She was too sweet to cause friction. Instead, she stayed close to him and gave him sniffies and kissies to calm down his meridians. Every time those beautiful pairs of numbers had submerged themselves in my life, it was always to give me a message from the ethers. It was always an opening to the gateway of enlightenment. It would be no wonder that she would follow him into heaven and that pair would be together forever.

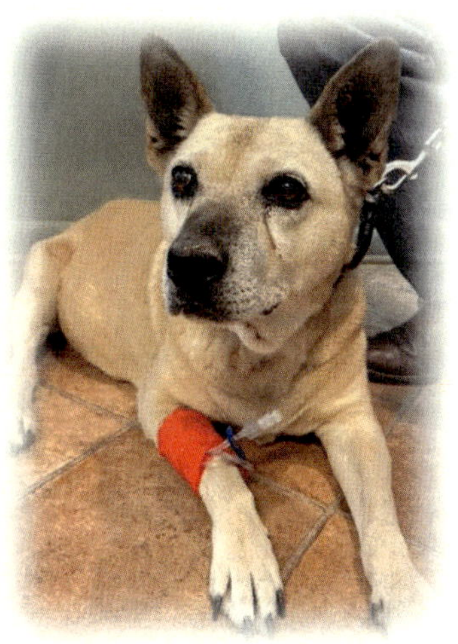

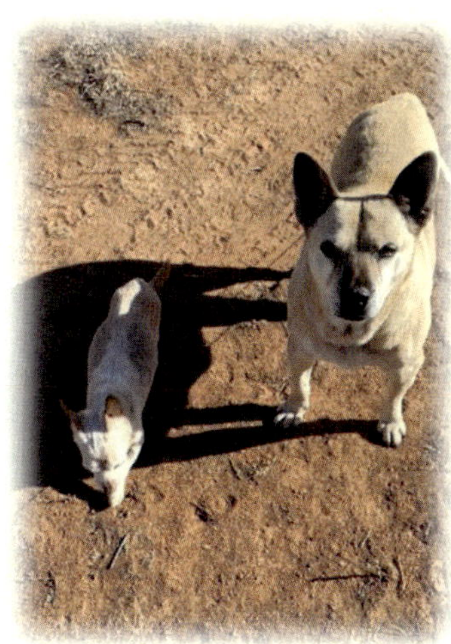

Surprisingly, my stepdad took it pretty well. He was sad, and he cried as she transitioned, but he seemed to bounce back quickly. He had witnessed more death in people and pets than any of us. That steal plate that protected his soft heart was built solid over many years. We got in the car and headed to the cemetery as planned. We spent a good while stopping by all the headstones and wall plates. We also spent time at his mom's gravesite. I knew it meant a lot to him. We even got to visit with my ex's father. They adored that man as well. He treated my parents like they were VIP members. It was nice to share good-hearted energy with him where he was laid to rest.

We made our last walkthrough and then jumped in the car to pick up some food and lottery scratch cards. We always enjoyed playing scratchies. We sat in the vehicle laughing and talking about all the good times we had with Selena. We even won a few bucks. We thought maybe it was a lucky day since it was 11/11. Or maybe, she was already sending us signs from the other side. Whatever it was, it kept the mood good. It also allowed us to accept her final moments on a higher vibration. We could've focused on losing her. But instead, we focused on the wonderful middle parts of growing with her.

Those are the remarkable gifts pets give us. They evolve with us, expand with us, and instill a lifetime of invaluable messages within us... so that when they're gone, we'll be okay. They inspire us to try new things, believe in new ways, and to persist even more in achieving our goals. When I brought Dipper into my life, I thought I was saving him. But really, he was saving me. He taught me so much about life and helped me remember the highs of my own.

Almost immediately after getting to know him, he began pointing out my most prominent features, which were compassion, healing, humor, writing, and creativity. By teaching me how to take care of him, he was showing me that I could carry on the lessons and utilize my strengths to help more Dippers. I had always been a person who was positively influential on many levels, so the rescue and natural therapeutic route for animals was already in my favor.

I knew I could always find a way back into entertainment if I really wanted to. Things constantly changed in that industry and people would forget, and rediscover, you overnight. But the more I looked into Dip's eyes, the more it became less desirable. I wouldn't be able to instantly replace the creative aspects of working in Hollywood, or the money that could be made in a single day from it. But I knew that because of him, I'd go on to contribute to something more important. And that wouldn't include a career path that was all about me. That business took every hour of every day, and required ultimate passion and dedication. Dipper did as well, and was so much more fulfilling. So, unless I got the chance to work on something that would be about him and benefit animals because of him – spreading compassion, curative awareness, and helping people heal from pet loss and bereavement – then the choice would be an easy one for me to make.

Since the color blue was such a strong representation of him, I knew that it was about the importance of self-expression. My Throat chakra had always been a struggle of mine physically. But I also felt the thyroid tenderness energetically. It wasn't that I had issues with saying what was on my mind. But in my field of work, you could get cancelled in a heartbeat. So, I played the game and was cautious in my posts, answered interviews carefully, and took certain roles and meetings to avoid being blacklisted. Yet, all that did was make me a puppet. I was who I was whether on the screen or on unemployment.

Add to that, I became progressively reserved due to being fully "shut-up" in my past relationship. I lost my confidence and focus, as well as my zest when I was in public. But since Dipper came into my life, I slowly began relearning how to be vocal again. Within months, I was getting back to a healthy mind state where I was remembering how fearless, endearing, and engaging I used to be. I was finally getting back to my authentic self and regaining my personality.

My dog sure did have a knack for getting through to me in so many ways. He'd been given up at 18 ½ years of age, and still carried on with vivacity. What a way to teach me how easy it was to forget the bad things that anybody had done to me, big or small, even if it happened five minutes ago. He showed me daily that life was too short to stay in a low-vibrating mode, and too close for anyone not to get along. I wasn't sure if his message was about forgiving others, or just about being okay with not holding on to what they did. But he showed me how easy life was by only remembering the good.

That kind of cognizance kept him from looking back. There was no need to. He had already been there and done that. His focus was solely on his present moment. When he had to move forward, he did so with simplicity and tempo… always going at his own pace and flow. And along the way, he showed me that I didn't have to do things on a wide scale. My mission wouldn't be less valuable because I rescued one senior dog at a time versus an organization that saved one every day. My intentions would fall into place as long as I stayed true to myself. Therefore, there was no point in rushing or forcing anything. The only place I needed to get to, and be… I was already there.

After Dip burst out of the ozone, he continued to help me grow and get better. All along, I thought there was a difference in the space he had been while in bodily form and the space he had transitioned to. After receiving signs from the other side, the totems, and the channeling through Bodhi, Lola, and recently Selena, I realized that he wasn't gone. He was still in doggy form and he still went to heaven. But instead of it being somewhere up in the sky, ***heaven was right where I was… with him in my heart.*** He was in his grandest form and highest light, and I was so happy for him. And since he was a part of my soul's architecture, I would always be walking parts of him.

We knew there was so much more to Dipper than just being a dog. He was Source Energy who enriched our humanness, spiritness, and Zen, while filling us with love oxygen. Through the process, one of his biggest revelations became the clearest: I wasn't any more stuck without him than I was before him. I missed him more than anything, and in large part, because of how good I felt when he was with me. He did such a great job of helping me remember what I was made of.

But I was lost long before he came into my life. I hadn't found what I wanted to do, where I wanted to go, or how I'd get anywhere. Yet, I had found him. For 169 days, he brought me back home, to my heart and core so that I could find myself again. In the time I traveled to the last few islands after his passing, I learned of the continual space of in betweens, and that *home wasn't a location.* ***Home was where my soul was.*** Dipper would still be Source Energy – and fuel us with love oxygen – and I would still continue getting better. The only difference was how I'd view his transformation and what plane we'd interact on.

His death had become personal. But like his life, it also became meaningful. I was slowly putting myself back together and remembering how to function again. I missed him, and smelled him in every flower. I breathed him in every breeze. I saw his radiance, and felt his warmth, in every ray of sunlight. I heard him in every beautiful poem and lyric. That was because he was another one of my soulmates. I never believed that there was just one person, a better half, that completed us. I didn't even believe that we were halves to begin with. That's how the concept had always been programmed in our minds.

But what if there were 2, 3, or 4, and in different forms? Those entities that come into our lives at different stages, each serving their own unique purpose? It's as if the scheduling of the Universe brings what's meant to be... when it's meant to be. Dipper was a pure example of that magic. Because of him, I learned that there were no age limits in who we shared immense love with. There were no timelines or measurements required to reach that level of harmony. Whether any of us connected when we were younger, and when they were puppies, or adopted them as seniors... they made us better. Whether they stuck around for fifteen years or for only a few weeks, they made us better. Because of them, we will go on to share love again, adopt and rescue again, work at something even harder, and do things in their names, memory, and honor. We will live out their best qualities. That will be their legacy.

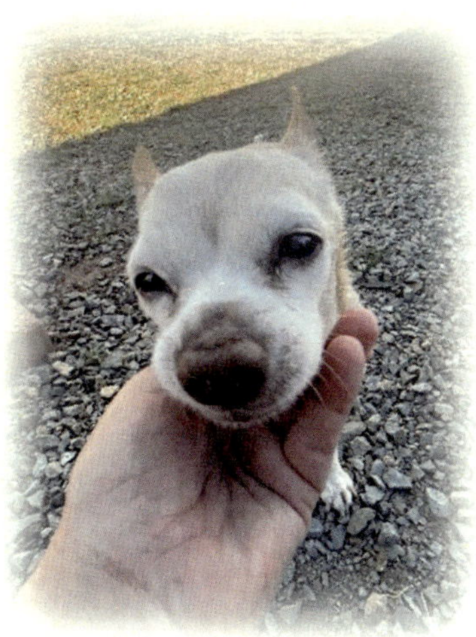

Thanksgiving was a day away and, like every morning, I woke up to see Dipper's face plastered all over one of my four picture boards. How I missed him. I always stayed glued to every image for a few minutes just reminiscing on the stories behind each photo. I felt a sense of peace that I didn't need to take him away from utopia so that he could save me. I was doing my part and it seemed to be working. I turned over to see Bodhi already leaning on his side, with his paw raised, so that I would rub his chest and belly. That little dude had it made. I said, "Good morning," to his scrunched little face and asked him if he slept well. Then we shared cuddles until Lola came up for air from under the covers.

As I'd stare into Bodhi's eyes, I always saw Charly. But I also started to see parts of Dipper. He never stopped leaning into my hands and picked up some of Dip's other traits and expressions. Lola was a whole new dog as well. She had become such a loving little girl. I knew it had to do with the same linking energy. They had both learned "You wanna go outside?" – "Who's here?" – "Thank you" – and "Grandma and Grandpa." I just had to say the words and they'd go nuts. I grabbed my laptop and cell phone from the bookshelf, and we headed towards the front door. I let the dogs out, and sat down at the kitchen table so that I could continue writing my story.

I had never been into huge celebrations for any holiday, so I wasn't looking forward to the extended weekend. I used to take that time to catch up and relax, but my mom was just the opposite. It was her specialty to bring people she loved together. I knew that meant I wasn't going to get much time alone in those four days, much less the following month, on into Christmas, and the new year. I decided to take full advantage of that last day of peace and quiet to see what my system came up with.

I sat there for a few minutes staring at Dip on my computer screen. I was always mesmerized by how much fur grew back on his ears and the grounding forces that exuded from his eyes. When I first got him, he was depleted. Within a day, he came back to life. He was more than a breath of fresh air; he was my air. I was so proud of how far the both of us had come together. As I was looking back on all that we accomplished, I thought to myself, "How lucky did I get?!"

I had spent so much of my time being fixated on moving that I didn't realize how incredibly blessed I was all along. I was in a safe, loving environment where I was given free range to do, be, and work on anything I wanted. I was living off the grid, in the middle of nowhere, away from people, masks, traffic, power lines, and pollution. I was surrounded by clean air, soft water, and magenta, lavender, and fiery orange sunsets. The globe was inundated in a collective health panic, racism was rampant, economies were plummeting, and people were losing faith. I wasn't around any of it. I was off social media and only on the internet to gather synonyms for my book. So, I was also far away from all the gossip.

I didn't own much of anything, wasn't bringing in an income, didn't have any jobs lined up, and didn't know how I'd live on my own again. Add to that feeling stuck, and without any drive. But my parents were my biggest fans and supporters. They offered their homes, their time, love, guidance, laughter, assistance, and financial backing. They never charged me a single dime in rent, utilities, or groceries. They actually paid my bills for almost a year and a half while offering me space to work through my issues. They did everything in hopes that I would get back on my feet again. Plus, they loved my dogs. They provided them with everything they needed, including top-tier food, health checkups, and medical treatments. Dipper, especially, cost them some money. He required natural homeopathic remedies, organic food and, at times, medical visits. None of that was cheap. They made changes to their houses and did whatever it took to make sure he was comfortable. They became grandparents. And, although maybe not in the way they had in mind, they were still every bit doting. When Dipper died, they also hurt badly.

My stepdad would drive his golf cart over almost every evening for dinner and we'd all share jokes and stories of the good old days. We'd crack up watching stand-up comedy shows. And on Friday nights, we'd go back in time and stream classic movies. We always had a blast building stuff at both properties and I'd chauffer him to the metro city for lunch and a few appointments. On the way back, we'd test our luck with scratchie tickets. All of us joined a weekly football pool, created amazing meals together, and took time to spoil Dipper.

I thought I wanted so much more for my dogs, especially Dip. Yet, after sitting with myself, and allowing my soul to bring things up to the surface, I realized that I was right where I was supposed to be. My mind, body, and spirit were so focused on relocating that I forgot how good we had it. There was no way I could've been in LA pursuing my long-gone acting career, working side jobs, hustling, and on everyone else's time, and still been able to give him everything. Nor, could I have grinded in a gym, trying to keep up to par with how that culture expected me to look, and still been able to share all those present moments with him.

After spending months working through my past and getting better with who I was then – what decisions I made then – and the outcomes from any of them – I was able to see the enormous advantages. Not having a job, being locked down, and having nothing else working for me allowed me to give every ounce of my time, energy, and attention to Dipper. I was able to love every part of him. I was able to improve his health, his livelihood, and elevate all the areas that kept him feeling like he was on top of the world. There was nowhere else I needed to be than with him. There was nothing else I had to do than to give him all of me.

I began to think that maybe all along I was preparing him for his next journey, because he blossomed almost immediately after coming into our lives. Maybe he found me so that I could strengthen him enough to make it through the atmospheric pressure and on to his next destination. Maybe he was giving me practice at handling the illusion of death so that I'd get better at it, and be more prepared for when my next senior soulmate comes for help. Maybe the exit out of his body appeared to be traumatic in order to teach me more about euthanasia. Maybe giving him the prescription medication that I knew would kill him, actually helped him to die faster. Maybe he had to show me how heartbreaking things could turn out when we think we're in control of anybody's destiny. Or maybe, it was a higher plan the entire time and everything happened exactly the way it was supposed to, and on perfect schedule, so that we could advance to the next level together. Maybe, just maybe, it was a final test to prove that we were meant to be.

If so, then thank God, Buddha, the Universe, the stars, sun, moon, sky, air, oceans, soil, and Mother Nature that I was the one who was given that assignment. There had never been anything more fulfilling or rewarding than sharing life with that little boy. Knowing that he went out a million times stronger, healthier, and happier than when I first adopted him showed me the real power of pure love and energy.

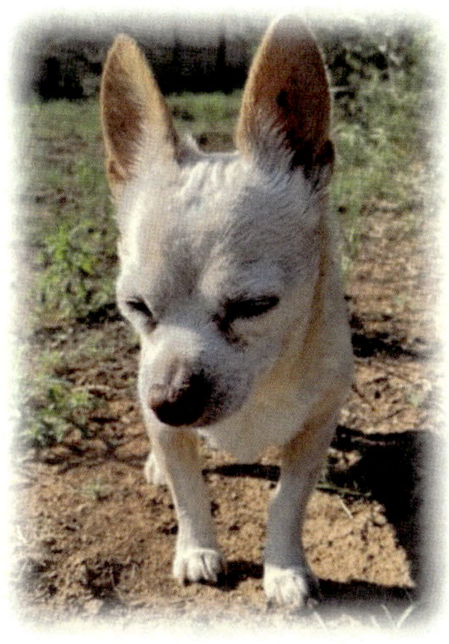

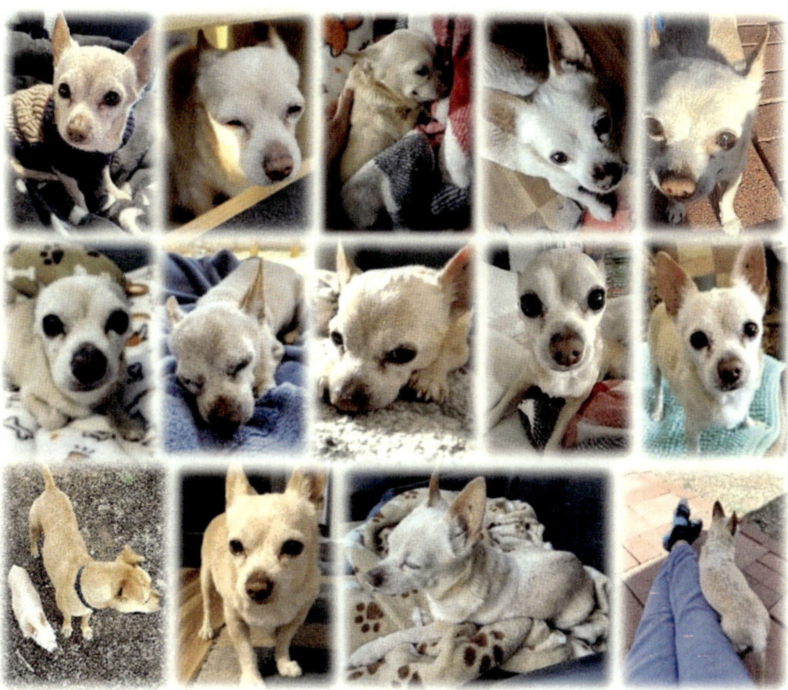

14
Divine Timing

It says a lot when we can choose to make a shift in our mindsets, especially when we've been hardest hit. Many times, the journey's so rugged that we don't even have any idea how we did it. I don't think sudden and unexpected change, and the uncertainty that comes with it, are ever welcomed. That includes all realms of death. Ends of tunnels are far from lit up and directions to find those openings are just as blurry and scary. Yet, isn't everything just a conduit to a different level and version of our higher selves? Every person, pet, place, thing, condition, absorption, response, and result – on both sides of the emotional spectrum – play the roles they do in evolving us into beings that can adapt, adjust, and move forward. Before long, we're breathing again and the rest of our surrounding ecosystems begin to ignite the flame into brighter environments. Doors start opening and, suddenly, we find our way to wholeness again.

I was beginning to resonate with the concept even more as my daily heart cracks started to close up... and the stitches, holding together what was left of my organ, were dissolving. The interactions between me and my parents also became much softer. I felt bad for complaining so long and being a walking firecracker. I could've blamed it on several things, including Goldie. But she was just being her authentic dog self. It was me who was a trauma pattern compounded with residual energy. I decided that, from then on, I'd remain nothing but gentle and lighthearted. There was still tension. They were who they were and had their own formulas, and I was still me. But there was no need to hang on to the arguments. We were all working towards the same goal... and that was happiness. In our own ways, we just wanted that for each other. I knew they needed me. They had provided me with everything my entire life, so it was my turn to repay the love. That meant doing all I could for them while I was still there, and getting them set up for when I wasn't.

The shift, and being fourteen weeks without Dipper, also took my focus away from the upcoming mediation. I had spent eight grueling months prepping for closure. Yet, I didn't care anymore. Dip was gone. Even the nightmares visited one night, and I didn't drown in the panic like I used to. I trusted the timing that something was coming to an end again. Maybe it was my dispute, or maybe it was simply brightening up my room.

A couple weeks earlier, I had covered the windows in both homes with plastic wrap to keep the freezing vibe out. I removed all the air conditioners except for mine, and packed them away in the outside storage. For some reason, I covered the entire unit with the blinds closed, leaving my room dark and grim. Dip would've never enjoyed a dreary room. So, I pulled out the heavy cooler and walked it over to the shed. As I was coming back, I was surprised to see an injured grasshopper on the bricks. It was almost winter and I thought they didn't make it that long. I knelt down to see why he couldn't walk and, surprisingly, he let me touch him. I asked what he needed so that he could jump. Yet, it didn't seem like he had any vigor left. So, I nudged him gently until he made it under the steps. I didn't want him to become a bird's breakfast. All of a sudden, he began to move on his own. I knew that it was because he felt safe enough to try again.

Another totem had come to remind me that we were all connected. I was also injured. I just needed to regain my internal stability so that I could take my own leap of faith. I walked back into the trailer and headed to my room. It was bright and lively once again. It reminded me how much fun Dipper and I, and all of the dogs, used to have in there. I was still sad, but the sun shined differently that day.

I was no longer concerned how the meeting would play out. If my ex and I weren't able to reach a reasonable agreement, then I just wanted it to be over. After going through what I did in the past four months, I realized that I didn't need to be compensated. I had already won. Because of him, I got to come into the lives of Charly and Tippet. And due to how things unfolded between us, I was able to meet more loves of my life and connect with my soul purpose. There wouldn't be any amount that could come close to that. So, in walking away, I was going to finally let go... and thank him instead of resent him.

Releasing the outcome of that case positively affected other areas of my life that had been on the backburner for many years. Since the early 2000s, I'd been trying to sell land in Colorado where I used to go tubing, fly fishing, and camping as a kid. We'd carry on the tradition into my teens, but once I was in college, it became rare to make the drive up there. My dad and stepdad, however, didn't hesitate in relishing in that pristine mountain ambience. They'd come back with plenty of fish to eat and tons of hilarious stories. That area was paradise for my dad. We dreamed of building a vacation home there one day. But after I left to LA, I never went back with him again. He died that following year. My mom and I held onto it for a little longer before putting it on the market. Interests came in, but we got low-balled with ridiculous offers.

Cut to eighteen years later and a pandemic. People began flocking in from all over. I got a call one day by a couple who invited me into town to discuss details. That meant I had to put on my happy mask before making the drive. Their home was designed with renewable energy and constructed in alignment with the coordinates of the sun, moon, stars, and the season's solstices. They had medicine wheels, kinetic sculptures, melodious windchimes, hand-made fairies in the trees, and a Peaceful Buddha Stone to sit on. They were extremely kind, cosmic, intelligent, and on a whole other spiritual level. Their ideas were remarkable, but they ended up having to pass on the sale.

As with most everything, there was something bigger than the purchase of that land. They decided to look for a place in Wyoming instead. Yet, they kept in touch through calls, and packages filled with astronomy, philosophical readings, and the introspective relativity of humanity. How lucky did I get? What a connection! What great timing! The awesome air must've reverberated because, not but a month later, it got sold to another heart-conscious, energy-aware family with some of the most sustainable and regenerative goals I had ever heard. Their vast knowledge and commitment to environmental and ecological cohesiveness for that entire community was the staple in turning over something so sentimental. My dad would've been proud and honored that a family would take over that place, create their own homestead, and love it just as much as he did.

The number "3" had been the best representation of me my entire life, so it would be no wonder why several things were falling into place. It was the last week of the turquoise blue month (12 → 1+2=3) and Dip's primary symbolic color. To many, it was holy. For me, the period represented accomplishment. It was about developed unity, trust, and divine connection. December was the twelfth page in the annual chapter of my story. As we were finishing up the final cycle of completion, everything that I was supposed to know in that moment… was coming together. The collection of air, souls, stars, suns, moons, messengers, reasons, and purposes would carry on to the next blank page and, once again, transition. Then, the rotation would begin all over again.

Aside from my picture boards and a few of Dipper's mementos, my room had been bare for almost four months. My dog's death had been such a shock to me that I couldn't be around anything other than similar hollowness. Yet, I had gotten better and was slowly filling the space back up with love and strength. I was starting to long for the essence and aroma that my spiritually awakening décor surrounded me with. I knew that I'd eventually unpack everything and get back to what I knew best. I would also get back to Bear and Spiffy.

They were two of my connective components that I hadn't stored away. I couldn't part with either of them because they were my family. Bear had been with me since crashing my vehicle into him at 14 young years of experience. His spirit would go on to take me through a metaphysical ride of my life and, in turn, help me to help others do the same. Then a cardboard smiley face entered seventeen light travels into it and elevated the dynamic even more. Since 2005, Spiffy went everywhere and did everything with me. He was my backbone, my pillar of strength, and my best friend. As silly as people thought he was when they first met him, he'd end up brightening their days more than ever. Before long, everyone wanted one of their own. Then Bear returned in physical form as my 43rd birthday present. He showed up just in time to remind me of my grounding forces, and to prepare me for what was ahead. Although we were alienated for the next three years, at least they both got to meet Charly and Tippet.

I knew people didn't quite get how I communicated with my plants and sacred belongings. They certainly couldn't grasp that I nurtured and talked to a stuffed animal and cardboard smiley face. Yet, they knew me. They may not have understood the energy behind my mental stimuli, but they'd still ask how to achieve the same upbeat aura and attitude. I always welcomed their views and continued showing them how to be their own scientific proof. I was lucky to have been taught the importance of imagination. It kept me from getting caught up in the outside noise. I also knew that meeting Bear as a kid was the precursor of how I'd connect on a deeper level as an adult.

I missed my formula with Bear and Spiffy. Our time had drastically decreased within months of my past relationship and even more since adopting my dogs. I felt bad that I hadn't spent closeness with them like I used to. They were placed on a nightstand in the corner of my bedroom just sitting there watching us play with Dipper. Then one day, I ran across something that made me realize there was nothing lost between us... especially love, presence, and togetherness. The Little Dipper was also known as "The Ursa Minor" (*The Little Bear*). Dip was my little bear and a mini version of my spirit animal the entire time! I had separated him from Bear and Spiffy, Bodhi, Lola, Charly, Tippet, Blue, Rudy, Fritz, Peaches, every totem, form, and experience. Yet, there was never any difference. Everything was connected to the whole. How I perceived and embraced one... would affect them all.

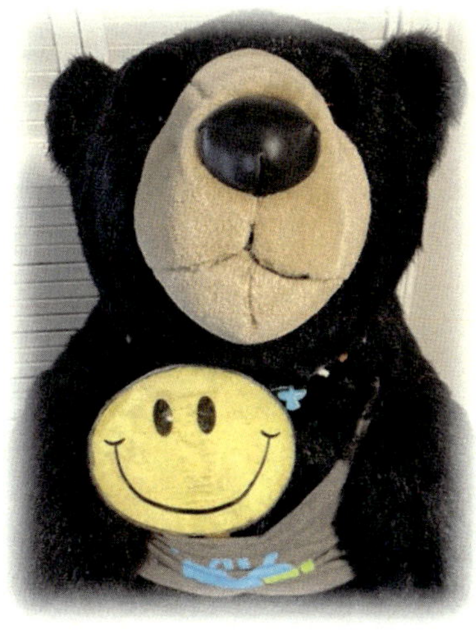

Christmas Eve arrived fast, and without any snowmen keeping watch outside. We hoped it wouldn't be another dry winter because that meant ice-cold winds and no runoff in the Spring. We were also praying that the blizzard gods would bombard us with flurries so we could stay in our jammies. The house was flashing with lights and ornaments. Plus, my mom made enough goodies as if we were bears getting ready to hibernate. Food was one of our favorite pastimes, which made the holiday one of our most enjoyable family gatherings.

The football games were also a key feature. My stepbrother and his daughter had made the trip up to the ranch to spend the evening with us, so it made it even more special. She worked for the local animal shelter and had a fond love for pets. She hadn't met Bodhi or Lola yet, so she was in for some melting. It was Bobee's second round at Christmas, but the first for Lolies with our family. We wanted to make sure they had the best experience ever. My mom even bought them gifts and conjured up some special treats.

I was trying my hardest to embrace Dip being with us in his own way, but I still wished that he was there in his fur body. I just wanted to watch him open his presents. I had dreamed of us spending that evening together in our own place somewhere far away. Obviously, it didn't turn out as planned. Yet, I was gaining comfort with it. I realized that Dipper might have not been able to handle the piercing weather. He loved the outdoors and I would've had to keep inside most of the time. That would've been torture for him. When I'd catch myself zoning off in those thoughts, I would smile at my family and act like everything was okay. No matter how far I had come, there was still emptiness without him.

We were just about finished unwrapping presents when my step-brother pulled out one last gift. It was fairly large and I didn't have a clue what it was. Then I opened the package and saw Dipper!!! He was on canvas! What a masterpiece of art he was! Words couldn't describe the feelings that came over me when I saw his brilliant little face. He looked so healthy and furry and at peace. I remembered the day I took that picture like it was yesterday. What a perfect way for him to show up. I cried lakes of tears for a few minutes, but it was a beautiful reminder of how much he had evolved with us.

I wiped off my smeared mascara and we toasted to the blessings. Then we watched a movie about a little boy who lost the spirit of Christmas because he wasn't convinced of Santa Clause. He ended up taking an interesting train ride to the North pole with other kids also struggling with self-doubts. They created friendships along the way and received messages that helped them discover their inner strengths. When they finally arrived, the gala was booming with music, elves, and a crew of restless reindeer. The kids were in awe, but the little boy was still skeptical. Then a silver bell broke off one of the caribou's leashes and rolled right to him. He picked it up, shook it, and nothing. So, he closed his eyes and allowed himself to believe; affirming out loud until he could hear the ringing. That's when the big man showed up to greet him! There was more to how everything unfolded. But what hit home, were the inspirational words the conductor hole-punched on each kid's ticket as they were boarding for the return trip. When he got to the little boy, his read "*Believe*."

Parts of the film were a bit weird, but those scenes were touching. It made me think that the little boy was dreaming, and the train was symbolic of his mind. He had to travel through certain stages so that he could get to a place of acceptance. That was the only way he could remain open to the magic. I pictured the conductor being the little boy's soul, and his purpose was to remind him what he knew all along. I had been given so many tools in those last four months; that would be one of the most powerful. As much as I'd always miss Dip in physical form, I had to believe that he'd always be with me. I had to believe that I'd get better and life would get better. I had to believe in myself fully. Mostly, I had to believe in the timing of everything.

I ended up sleeping straight through the night. It was nice to rest so deeply. The next morning, I laid there thinking about who I used to be before moving back to New Mexico. Things had dramatically shifted, so I was always going to miss a part of who I was and what I identified with. I didn't like starting over, but at least I'd get to try again with more experience and a higher level of consciousness. I had no idea what was in store, but I had my book to help me move forward. I also knew that me, Bodhi, and Lola would go on to help more amazing senior pets receive love to the fullest. I believed that.

As I glanced at my 1st and 2nd Moons nuzzled up together, I saw how great they were for each other. They became besties with their own personalities, and shared almost everything. Lola was like Poison Ivy when we first got her and just as combustible as a bottle rocket. Yet, her survival mode was only temporary. Who knew what she went through that caused her to be so territorial? It took that little girl nine months to begin trusting us. She still barked at air and was a spitfire towards Goldie. But it was nice to see her gain enough security to show her vulnerabilities. She'd roll around on her tummy, sneak into my blankets, and lick the moisturizer off my face and water off my legs. Plus, she couldn't kiss enough. That was her specialty. She'd chum up to my parents and swindle them out of their food, and then hump her bed right in front of us. Like Bodhi, she stuck to me like glue. And, out of all the dogs, she was the most playful and best behaved.

The more I looked at her, the cuter she became. I didn't have such animosity towards her for how she acted in the past. Maybe that was because I wasn't so immersed in it. I actually began to care about her, and learned to work with her uniqueness in ways I would've never thought possible. Seeing her come out of a protective shell was beautiful. It made me proud to have given her a second chance and share such great experiences. I couldn't imagine us returning to our former rift. She was a spicy little jalapeno with the hugest heart. It just took a bit longer to get to a place where she could share it with us.

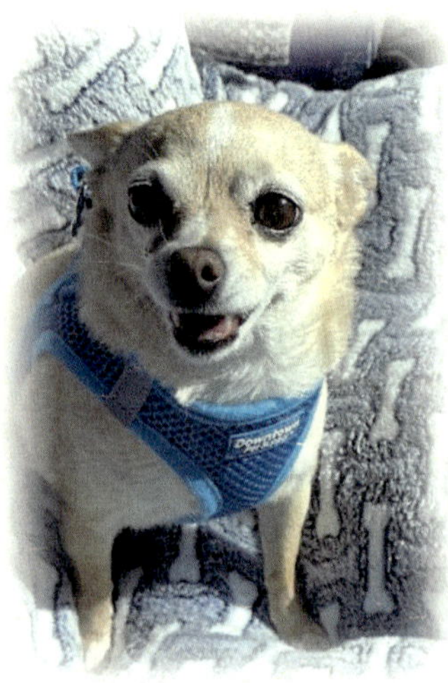

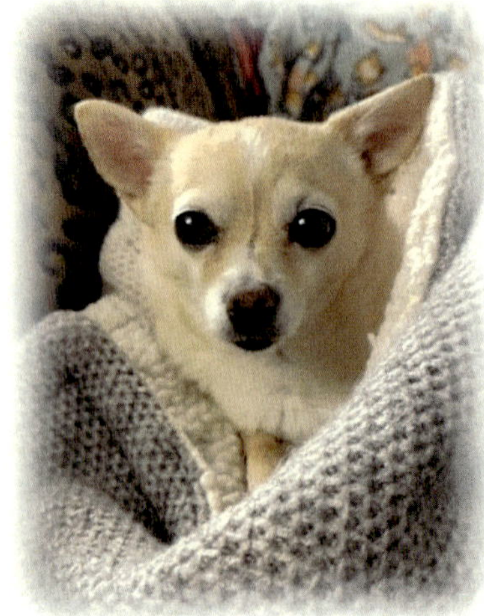

Surprisingly, Bodhi started getting a little feisty. Sometimes I had to wonder what got into him. Then I remembered that Goldie had been picking on him for a year. She never hurt him; she just wanted to play. Yet, she was much bigger, so her form of play was too rough. No matter how frustrated I got with her, she never hurt any of my dogs. She'd actually submit and make them think they were champions. She rolled them a few times in the weeds and dirt, but never dominated them with aggression. When Dipper was alive, she always stayed close and watched over him. I saw how it made him feel like a King. She was irritating most of the time, but was a spiritual asset in so many other ways. I thought about how she was there for me when I moved in with her and my parents. I felt bad that I had changed towards her and that our relationship was different. But I knew she didn't. She still loved us with all of her heart and would be there for us no matter what. That was the gem she truly was.

I had to say that Goldie played a role in Bodhi standing up for himself and being a little bad ass. I wanted to buy him a bomber jacket one time, but learned that he wasn't up for any kind of clothing. He tried to bite my face off when I put a sweater on him. He hated to be smothered, detested getting his nails cut, and his butt was still off limits. We had to respect his space and boundaries. Regardless of how tough he'd act, he was still a whiner and a love bug who followed me around like a shadow. He'd clutch my arm tightly with his paw so that I wouldn't stop rubbing him. That was his way of telling me to please never leave him. He was such a compassionate little creature, and soft and calming as a mix of vetiver and chamomile essential oils.

I could've called him a Zen Meister because of the intuition, harmony, and wisdom he embodied. The dude was a collection of Heart, Third Eye, and Crown chakras, and the 528 Hz love frequency who came in the form of four paws, fur, and fourteen pounds of amazement. In so many ways, he brought our family balance. He was so playful and so innocent, and absorbed every ounce of love that we gave him. I knew Bodhi was special when I first laid eyes on him, but I had no idea the gift he would turn out to be. Because of him, we were able to connect to a deeper level of gratefulness. Because of him, Dipper got to experience the highest part of all of us.

I remember how scared he was when I first met him. I hated that people had hurt him, but he was increasingly flourishing. We offered him the stability to live freely and trust us deeply. He turned 4 years of awesome experience on the first of the month and we celebrated the amazing pack leader he had become. Just like Dip, he got a special entrée, cake, and four candles to wish upon while we sang to him.

He would always carry a fear of abandonment, but it wouldn't stop him from sacrificing himself for the better of the collective. I knew he'd take a back seat again and play a different role to make sure we could help another senior family member. That was how unselfish that little boy was. The spiritual soul energy experiencing his doggy earth body was that beautiful. Bodhi was my superhero. Never could I imagine life without him. Yet, as celestial as he was, I knew I would also lose him someday. No matter how prepared at the time, it will be just as devastating... and the process will begin once again.

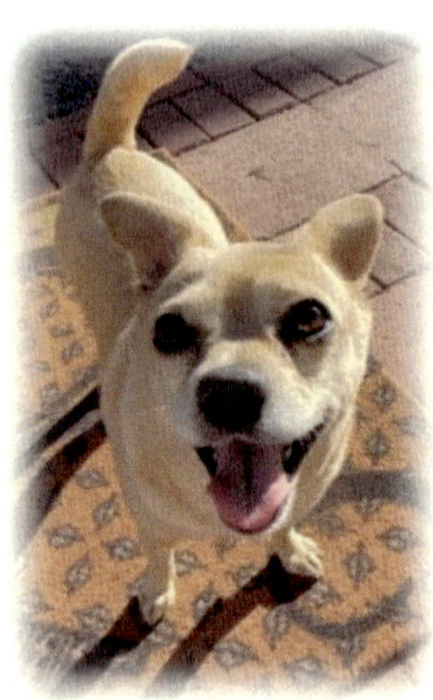
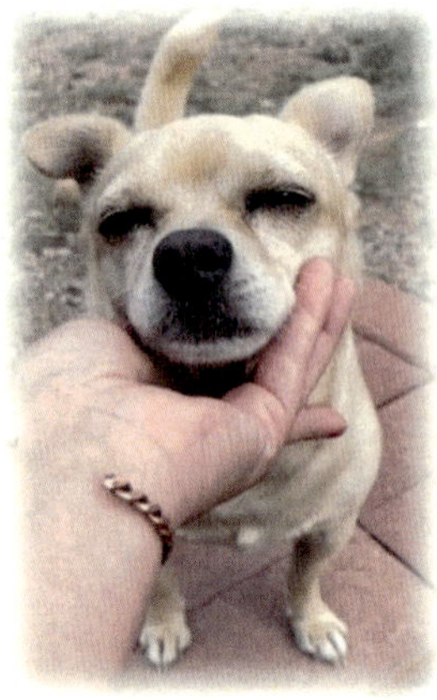
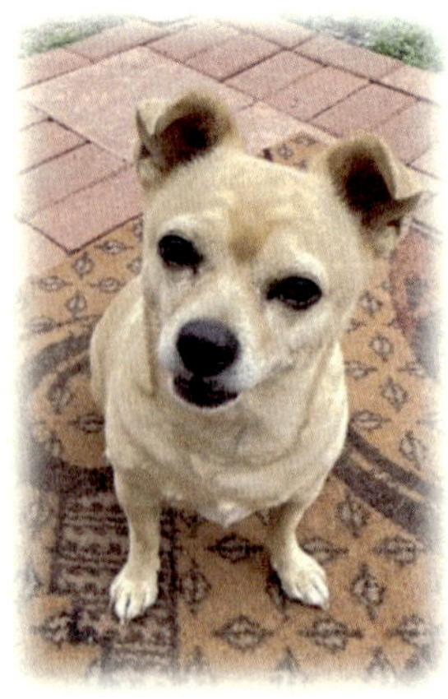

It made me wonder if anything ever fully gets completed in life, or if we just get to a place of peace. After dealing with Dipper's death, and going back in time to heal my past, I realized that everything was one continuous story filled with cycles of last lines on last pages in last chapters... just like the twelve rotations the moon makes around the earth annually. Nothing ever stops, it just changes direction. Pasts don't end, they just get remembered differently. Physical bodies, conditions, and connections don't die. They just shift forms. We have the power to rewrite the story so that it's a more pleasant one.

I had traveled in and out of six stages of healing most of my life and continuously dealt with ongoing stories of pain and struggle. The hardships got worse and the deaths got more painful. It wasn't until I began releasing and forgiving on island #7 that I would get to a place of acceptance and peace with my past and the current me. I was able to begin closing what I could of previous chapters so that they wouldn't ruin my new ones. It would be no wonder that the number "9" was so connective with the cycles of life and death... release, forgiveness, acceptance, peace... and completeness.

1. Shock
2. Anger
3. Guilt
4. Sadness
5. Emptiness, Lostness
6. Fear
7. **Release, Forgiveness**
8. **Acceptance**
9. **Peace**

I don't know if anybody ever fully gets over the loss of a pet, or anyone they love, for that matter. I do believe, however, that we have the choice to release ourselves from the attachment to their final moments, outcomes, and how we could've done our parts differently. We deserve that comfort, especially since we'll continue on with pieces of our hearts missing.

I knew my dog was going to die that day. I saw it that morning on his face and the way he lifted up his head to tell me. I just didn't know it would happen like it did. I wish I had a magic wand to change that whole scene ending and relive it another way. Yet, that wasn't his destiny. All I had was the beautiful middle to share my energy with and the opportunity to work through my grief.

As you've just read, there hasn't been anything easy about the process. Fortunately, I was able to come to a place of acceptance where I could view the changes of the wind more positive, rather than being curses. I was able to see that my little Dipper brought me back home, to my roots, so that like a flower, I could regrow in fruitful soil instead of being smothered in mud. I would always miss him, and always miss us in the formula that I had attached myself to. There wouldn't be anything like having him back in fur, paws, and long wet kisses. Thankfully, I was learning how to embrace his new structure and location, so that I could continue our beautiful narration. Because of Dip, I was going to be proof that recovery was possible.

He was a consistent flow of unconditional love, the gateway to enlightenment, and the glue that brought everything meaningful back together. He wasn't a half moon. He was a full moon. And although he wasn't as physically strong as my other dogs, he made up for it in so many other wonderful ways. The time I was blessed to share with him was more rewarding than I could've ever envisioned. Thank goodness we came to each other when we did. He was my all, my prana, my soulmate, my bloodline, my heartbeat. He was everything that I needed, and I was everything for him. There was no question that Dipper and I were both going places. We just needed each other to help get us there. Him and I hit the jackpot together. In fact, we all did. So, although our forever may have only appeared to be a season and a half, in the end of no ends, it was just another cycle of completion. We'd continue on because he paved the Peace Way. Dipper "Veteran" Moon would always be our little blueprint. 💙

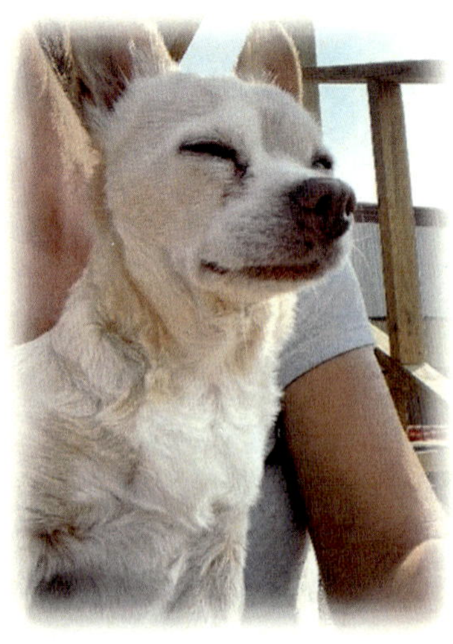

The holidays came and went, and it was time to close out the year's cycles of startups and finishes. I was a pet parent who had lost three fur children within twelve moon rotations; the last one enough to die for. I could've felt sorry for myself and looked at the year as my absolute worst. Instead, I saw it as my absolute best. How could it not be? I met Dipper... and for 5 ½ months we got to share our best parts with each other. All of my dogs were able to share in the ethereal experience and all became better from it. How blessed were we?!

It was the 31st and four months to the exact date that he transitioned, transformed, and transcended. As painful as parts of it still felt, the timing was magical. I didn't know if it was a Higher Plan, Divine Order, luck, fate, or karma. I just knew that the choice was a power I had learned through nine stages of healing, and consciously shifting my mindset about final moments. Hence, my heart, my mind, meridians, chemicals, and energy in motion improved. My adrenal glands still needed some help, but the aches in my body almost completely disappeared. That's what happens when you can work through your grief and begin shifting shit into sunshine, heartbreak into harmony, and loss into love. Instead of asking myself, "Why do dogs die?"... I chose to see it as, "Why do dogs come into our lives?"

What a beautiful exchange of energy I was able to share with my little boy. How I miss him. How I will always miss him. How I will always miss all of them...

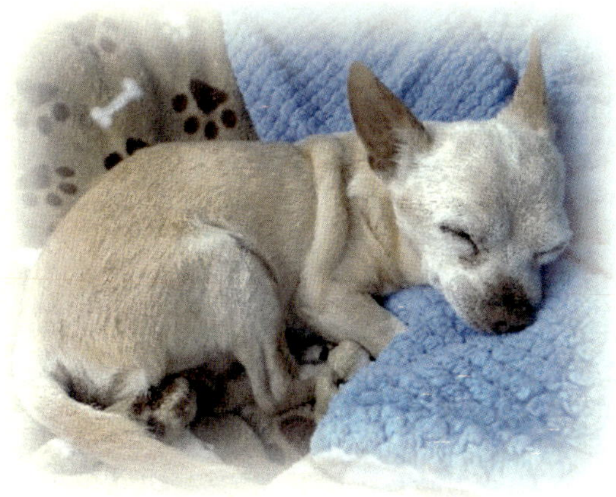

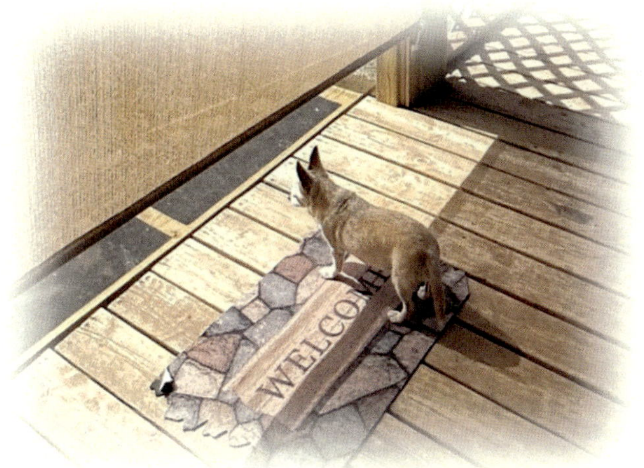

Always and Furever...

Bonus: 15
The Afterglow

Talk about timing. Every occurrence and person in my life played a role in bringing me back to dogs. Then, with each new furry connection and encounter, I was collectively led to Dipper... and aligned with my life mission of giving senior rescues the best experiences they'll ever have for the rest of the time they have left. As challenging as the first four months of my recovery were, they were also some of the most rewarding. Not only did I begin healing my past, but I was able to move forward with less sadness. I still had days where I questioned whether or not I was cut out to do the work with senior animals that I had felt fulfilled in doing. I didn't know if I could watch another gentle helpless creature take a painfully turbulent exit again. I knew I had a gift in bringing animals back to life and to a stage where they would ultimately thrive. But the length of time you get to share unconditional love with them is never long enough. That's tough to digest and even tougher to have a piece of your heart ripped out so often. Then, after seven months of gradually progressive feel-good days, another special little guy came to me!

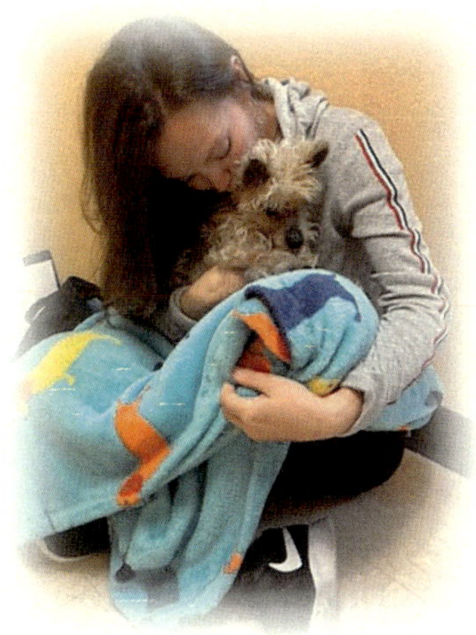

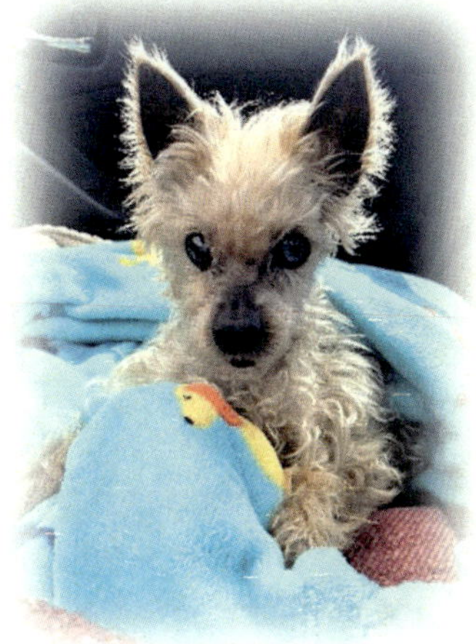

Never did I think I'd be ready to undertake another soulmate so soon. Yet, once I met him, I instantly loved him. He was a 15-yr-young Yorkie who had been found as a stray crossing one of the busiest streets in the city. He was skin and bones, almost fully blind and deaf, had a red, raw bald spine, matted fur on his limbs, leather black ears and nose, a serious eye injury, a heart murmur, kidney and thyroid issues, showed signs of cognitive impairment, and had an emergency surgery to remove a mass on his jawline the day before adopting him. He also had no testicles. So, at some point, he was in someone's care enough to neuter him. On his records, he was listed as, "Not an adoptable candidate." After reading that info, I knew he was perfect.

He would be our 4th Moon and go by "Cosmo" from then on. Just like Dipper, he immediately adapted to our loving surroundings and began an organic whole food, non-synthetic healing journey. His transition was just as miraculous and magical, as he returned to optimal health, weight, and the youthful spirit that he still had plenty left of. His melt-worthy personality would shine through by the way he'd playfully rub his head in the beds, dig through his blankets, scope out our moves, chomp on watermelon, run around outdoors, explore the hallway, and lay on his side while lifting his paw so that we'd rub his chest and belly. His only disability was not being able to fully see. Yet, you would've never known because he got where he needed to go. After starting weekly acupuncture, he began regaining some of it back, as well as his hearing. Aside from a bout with head pressing, and a day of two grand mal seizures that we thought were due to wildfire smoke and heat, he showed no cognition issues. He was filled with the confidence and willpower as that of an active Solar Plexus. Plus, it was amazing how his Heart & Root chakras would flourish by the way he understood the closeness and grounding I shared with him.

We were approaching his 4th month with us when, one morning outside, he had a seizure in my arms. It seemed mild, but I still asked him to let me know if it was time. Within ten minutes, he had another one. Then he became severely disoriented and paralyzed on his left side; falling on his face while racing in every direction. It was shocking how sudden he went from amazing to non-functioning, especially when things were going so well. I was crushed, but didn't want him to go through what Dipper did. So, I panicked.

I got his little deflated self ready and drove him into town. By a few miles in, it happened again. We finally made it to the emergency animal hospital and life flashed before both of our eyes in seconds. His became despondent as he began his exit. Mine were devastated. He laid in my lap for his last breath and fell into his deepest of sleeps.

It was absolutely awful to hold him while motionless. Knowing that I would never again share life with him in bodily form, smell his baby soft aura, or create any new and fun formulas together was horrible. I loved Cosmo more than anything. Yet, somehow, I knew we'd always be deeply connected on every level. He may have already been in a *better place* with me. But now he was free. Now, he could finally see.

Just like all of my dogs, he shared meaning, gratitude, fulfillment, and invaluable messages to make me an even better human. Because so, I would carry on his legacy. I had been dealt that card back-to-back and was reaffirmed that we can give them every ounce of our love, the best healthcare, top nutrition, an oasis of comfiness, safety, protection, trust, freedom, and do everything to keep them alive... and we still won't be able to force our pet's destiny to be what it isn't.

I began working through my guilt of ending his life so fast, and processing the sadness and emptiness without him. I kept thinking how in the world did he make it on the streets alone. Then I'd thank that same world that he made it to me. He was another beautiful part of the story... and another reason to continue with my soul purpose. It was such a blessing to have gotten that time with Cosmo. How lucky was I that he chose me to love all of him... and prep him for his grand entrance into the High Land? Thanks to Dipper, that became possible.

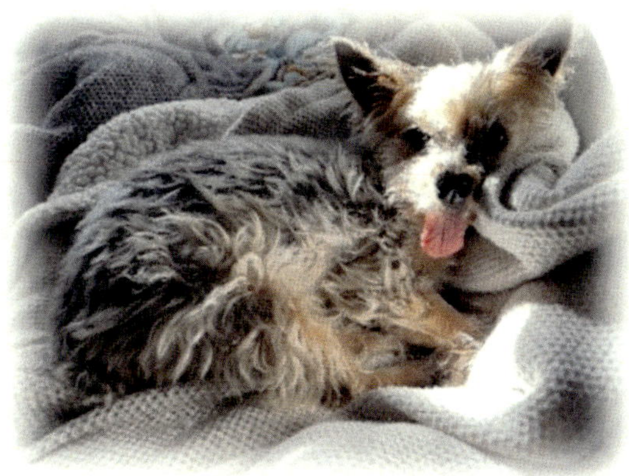

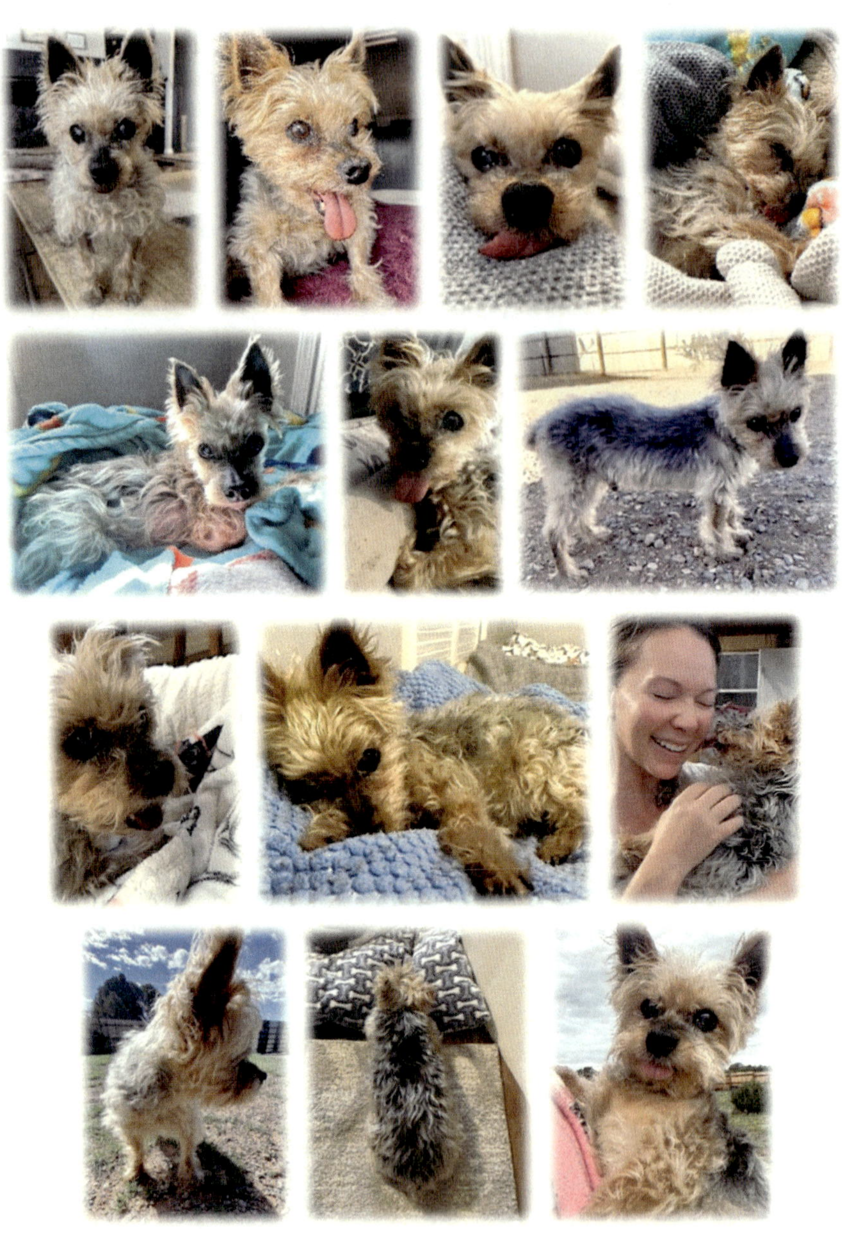

Cosmo "Cozzy" Moon

♥

Bonus: 16
The Spirit of Life

They say that with death, comes birth – with endings, come beginnings – and with closings, come openings. Yet, grief had felt like one ongoing wavelength of pain. It wasn't until Dipper's transition that I was able to understand that it was okay to feel that way. Coming to terms with loss was a process. And from my shared experience with him, I was able to embrace a lifetime of transitions, including the most recent with my precious Cosmo. Don't get me wrong, I hated myself for failing him by not trying to save him. But as with all other cycles, the Universe didn't allow me to stay stuck in that frequency for long.

Three months after Cozzy's passing, a tiny 16-year-old fella named "Walter" crossed my path. Like all times before, I wasn't in a position to bring in another family member. But I was learning that things didn't usually go as planned. I decided to drive out the next morning to meet the little guy, especially since he was a replica of Dipper.

He was such a beautiful, sweet Chihuahua. But his shivering skinny frame and hair loss on his neck, spine, tail, and hind legs indicated some issues. He also had oil and tar on his head, and seemed dazed as to why he was there. I couldn't tell if he was deaf or just not paying attention to me. However, it was clear that he wanted out of that facility. He'd been there for twenty-one days with no full exam, blood tests, or treatment. All they knew was that he had been confiscated, thought to have minor tarter and kennel cough, and wasn't neutered. Within minutes, I noticed something peculiar with his hairless penis. When I looked closer, I realized that it was his tail that was tucked up into his abdomen... and Walter was actually a little girl!!!

Shelters did their best, but it was hard not to judge. I was still thankful to have connected with her there. I was also able to take her home because they suddenly found a spay scar and what seemed to be a canine tooth pulled. So, at some point, she was in the hands of someone who cared, or placed in a shelter earlier in her life.

We immediately headed an hour back to the animal clinic. She ended up having pneumonia, a low thyroid, and a super high count of white blood cells and lymphocytes. Yet, her exam, blood work, and x-rays didn't show organ failure, a murmur, enlarged heart, fluid, cognitive issues, heartworm, ringworm, or ehrlichiosis. She was going to need a dental cleaning (all canines still intact), and had a possible cataract. But I hadn't dealt with pneumonia or chronic infections before. So, it would be a learning course. In fact, a few fosters I knew had lost their rescues to the same lung condition that week and it was heart-wrenching. I had to take a chance to give her a chance though. She was perfect and I believed in her to the fullest. From that moment on, she'd become our 5th Moon and go by the name of "Spirit."

I instantly saw the light of Dipper and Cosmo in her radiant eyes. I knew she was going to be the continuation of the love story, essence, and influence of all my beloved dogs who carried the torch before her. And like them, she'd also bring in her own unique glow. From the sun to the moon, the air to the ocean, the sky to the soil... she'd become the root that connected their beautiful cycles infinitely in my soul. She would be my kin, my oxygen, my everything... and another furever soulmate. I had no doubt that she'd progress and thrive like never before. And as long as we would have together, we would share our best parts with each other. We'd fully be in the present moment just like Dip and Cozzy taught me. Welcome home "Spirit Moon!" May the rest of your time here... be the best you've ever had!

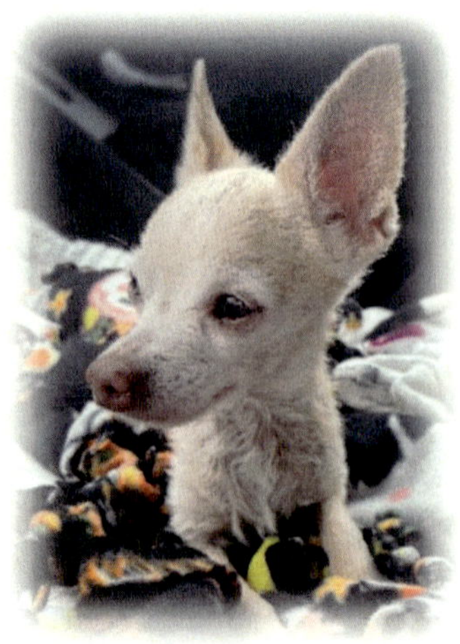

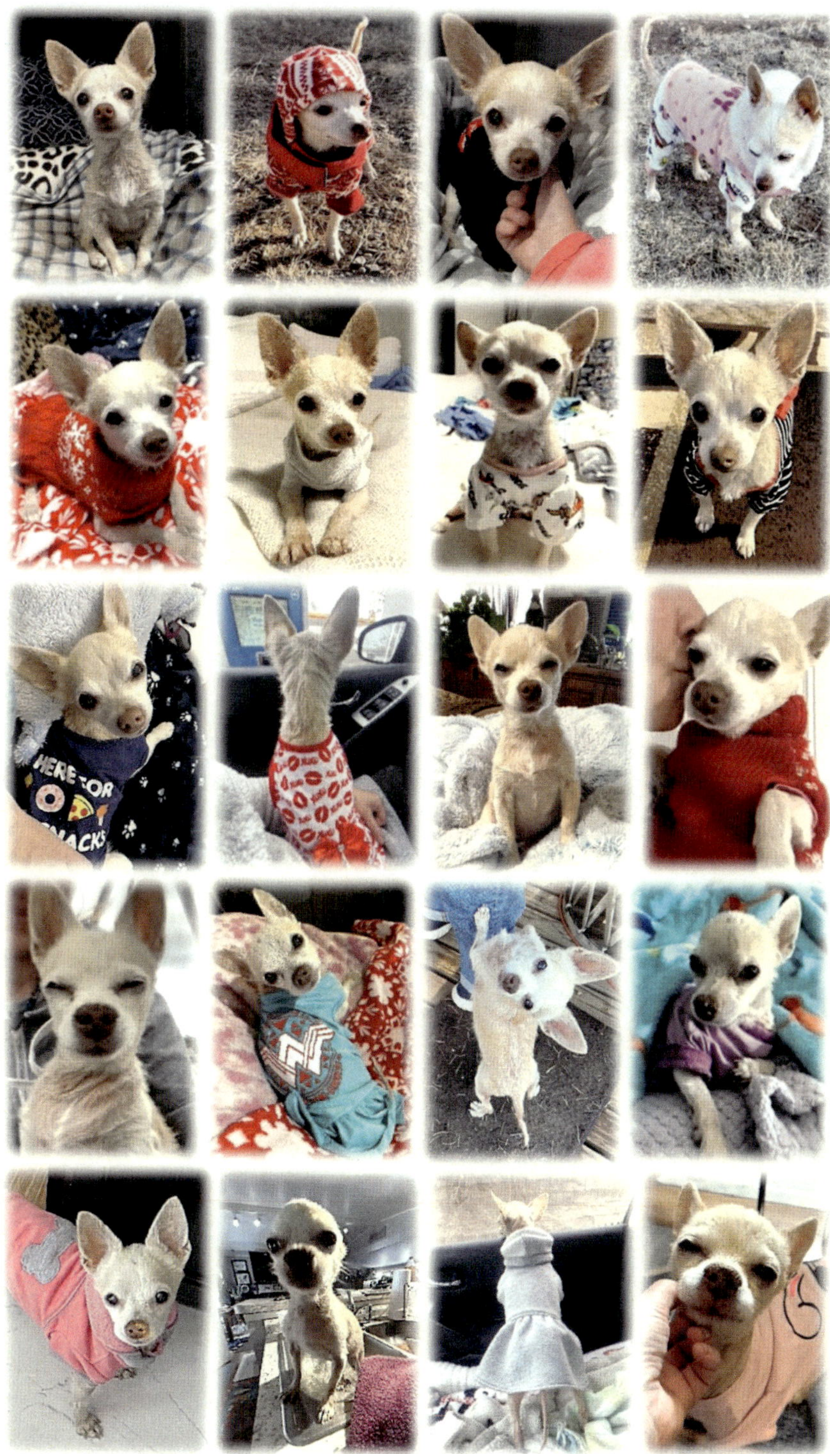

In loving memory of our soulmates

♥

References

~ The ownership and rights of all the photographs belong to the author, and were taken with her cameras. The photos of Charly and Tippet were taken when both dogs shared residency with the author, when she shared ownership of the dogs, and when the dogs were in her full-time care. Both pictures of Blue were taken when he was on the premise where the author shared residency, and when he spent time with her there.

~ The ownership and rights of the pencil drawing on the last page belong to the author. The drawing was created by artist, Edgar Flores.

~ Permission has been granted to the author for the usage of names, texts, and emails of, and sent from, her friends including Maria Reich (The Pet Health and Nutrition Center) on pg. 171.
https://www.pethealthandnutritioncenter.com/

~ Photo of Bodhi Moon – Pg. 69
Santa Fe Animal Shelter & Humane Society / Intake name: Cody / Shelter photo
https://sfhumanesociety.org/

~ The Bodhi Tree Bookstore – Pg. 75
Founded in 1970 / 8585 Melrose Ave., West Hollywood, CA 90069
https://en.wikipedia.org/wiki/Bodhi_Tree_Bookstore

~ Tuesdays With Morrie (Book) – Pg. 165
By Mitch Albom
https://www.amazon.com/Tuesdays-Morrie-Greatest-Lesson-Anniversary/dp/076790592X

~ Katydid / Moving Leaf Bug – Pg. 175-177
https://spiritanimaldreams.com/katydid-symbolism/
https://spiritanimalsandsymbolism.com/katydid-spiritual-meaning-symbolism-and-totem/
https://naturallycuriouswithmaryholland.wordpress.com/2013/08/09/clean-antennae-necessary-for-sensory-perception/

~ Surviving Death (2021 Netflix Docuseries) – Pg. 198
What happens after death? / Near-death, Reincarnation, Paranormal Phenomena
https://www.netflix.com/title/80998853

~ Guns N' Roses (Music Band) / "November Rain" (Song Lyrics) – Pg. 199
Writers: Darren Reed, Duff McKagan, Izzy Stradlin, Matt Sorum, Saul Hudson, Axl Rose
https://www.songfacts.com/lyrics/guns-n-roses/november-rain

~ Ursa Minor / Little Bear (The relation to the Little Dipper) – Pg. 220
https://en.wikipedia.org/wiki/Ursa_Minor

~ The Polar Express (2004 Animated Film) – Pg. 222
Director: Robert Zemeckis
Writers: Chris Van Allsburg (book), Robert Zemeckis & William Broyles Jr. (screenplay)
https://www.imdb.com/title/tt0338348/

~ Number "9" Numerology (The Concept of Completion) – Throughout the entire book
https://www.numerology.com/articles/about-numerology/single-digit-number-9-meaning/

A Little About Me and Why I Wrote This Book

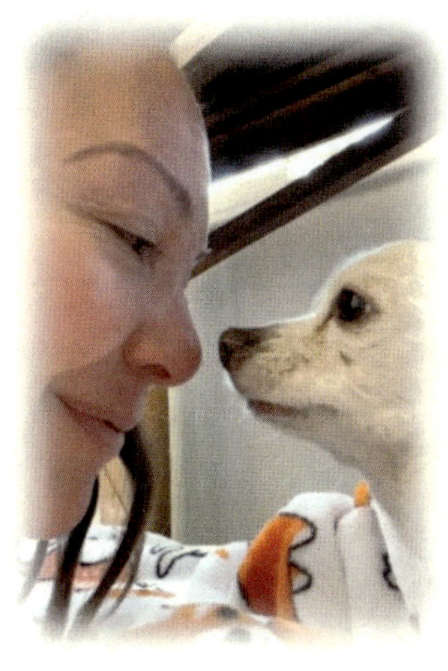

I've done and been a lot of things in life, met some phenomenal animals and people, and gained a great deal of wisdom from the highs and hardships. I grew up in New Mexico, graduated from college in state, and spent almost twenty years in LA working as an actor, host, model, and writer. I'm lucky to have booked some cool commercials and awesome tv and film projects. I'm also very proud to have written an amazing motivational book, *"Been There, Done That... now doing MORE!"* and a poetry piece titled, *"Love Art."*

In the acting profession, it can take plenty of side jobs to keep you going until getting to a level of steady booking. I certainly hustled my fair share trying to get there. Yet, one thing that was always consistent was my free-spirit thinking. Since I was a young adult, I had been fascinated with mind expansion, self-help, and natural healing methods. I was like a modern-day hippy absorbed with crystals, techniques, creativity, and spirituality. In addition to healthy nutrition and exercise, those tools were what kept me as mentally balanced as possible.

Showbiz can be a tough business. It takes confidence, drive, talent, and a steel-coated plate to be able to withstand the constant rejection. I started that ride as a self-assured, fun, loving, kind, person with a huge heart and warm personality. Eventually, I got worn down and began considering less stressful jobs... all the while, waiting for that once in a lifetime role. What kept coming back to me was my natural gift to uplift. I was always drawn to providing emotional wellness. Before I knew it, I began dabbling in energy work and life coaching. By 2014, I added *"Moon"* to my name and found myself helping others, and writing self-empowering stories, more than being on tv and in movies. In 2021, I also legally added *"Star"* to my name to begin the second part of my journey.

Like many performers. I fell into other occupations. Yet, I would've continued motivational and healing work in tandem with any pursuit. It wasn't until reconnecting with dogs in my early 40's that I was able to accept and be proud of the direction my career took. They became my focus and purpose, and navigated me to a special little rescue who brightened up my world and made all things meaningful. Life with him was a type of fulfillment I couldn't explain; so much that I knew he was my calling. Then he died, and I didn't know how to go on without him. I had to find a way to breathe and take the next step forward... and that's how *"Why Do Dogs Die?"* evolved.

In the beginning, I was trying to cope with the loss and heartbreak from the way he made his exit. I also think I just wanted people to cry with me and tell me how sorry they were. As time went on, I realized that there was so much more to our story than his closing moments. We shared a beautiful middle space where we grew and got better together. Then I began to see how indicative it was of life. I had spent so much of my adulthood attached to the sting of other unfavorable outcomes; never the in-between essence and substance of what got me there.

It was embarrassing to confront myself for what I allowed and how my life temporarily turned out. But it happened the way it did and it led me to a dog that pulled me out of the quicksand. In body and in spirit, he began taking me through a healing journey back in time so that I could find relief with other parts of my past. I started forgiving myself for making decisions that went against my gut, for thinking I could've done things differently, and for believing I had control over destinies. I was also regaining my personal power by letting go of thinking others were liable for where I got rerouted. All of my beloved dogs played a role in bringing me back home, to my heart and soul, so that I could find myself... and the core of my happiness. And because of Dipper, I began finding ways to be okay with the cycles of completion, including his.

I don't think anyone gets over a pet, or a loved one, for that matter. I also don't think we ever fully get closure, or the answers we need, in order to move on from the situations that hurt us most. However, we do deserve peace and comfort. Grief isn't something that clears up overnight. I definitely still struggle and will hurt in some way forever. But I've been brought to my life mission. No matter the challenges, I will continue to get better. Dipper taught me that. I adopted him at 18 ½ years of age and he was living life to the fullest... so why shouldn't I?

Today, I can say that I made it out of the low-vibing frequencies with gratitude, knowingness, and clarity of my soul quest. I went from loving the idea of being a public figure... to spreading uplifting, natural healing energy outside of the glamour. I've shifted my intentions to helping save senior shelter animals, and I've loved it even more. By sharpening what I've learned and constantly expanding my curative openness, I've been able to give these appreciative beings the best lives they've ever had. Thank goodness for Charly and Tippet. They were the first to show me that age, history, health status, and departure weren't factors. It was about the eternal connection instilled within us... and the value of the present moment in the temporary time anyone is here to visit.

It's been an honor to map this mending process through my little dog's divine light. That's what a special vital force he was. That goes for all of my darlings and the awareness they've brought to adoptions and rescues. In the time this book took to get published, I saved, fostered, and re-homed even more including a sweet, severely emaciated, neglected, deaf, semi-blind, flea and tick infested, 17-yr-old Terrier mix I named "Digo" ("Indigo"). He became my 6th Moon, but I didn't feature him because my piece only covers the first four months of my healing path and touches on the following two years with Cosmo and Spirit. But trust that he, and all those I got into safe, loving environments, benefited from the enriching aspects that my timeline of dogs infused me with.

You will travel your routes, have unique experiences with your pets, and contend with your own coping processes. Hopefully, mine can be symbolic of life in general. No matter the hardship, whether it be losing a dog, or losing a job – losing a marriage, or losing a child – it will be up to you to decide how to reconnect with your inner harmony. There is no timetable to rehabilitation; there are only the choices we make in releasing ourselves from the pain. You might not bring another soulmate into your life right away, or ever. And that's okay. My wish is that my journey helps you remember the good parts of yours, so that you can move forward with some cushion in your hearts. Maybe one day, you'll change your mind and have the strength to share true love again with one of the many deserving animals still out there. This book did that for me. And because so, it would always be a tribute to my little soulmate.

To all of my soulmates...

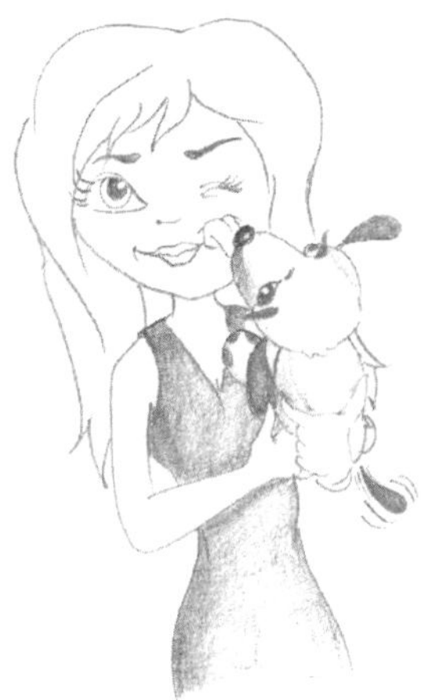

Second chances aren't just for pets; they're also for us.
If you can foster a shelter animal, please do. If you're in a position to take on the love, companionship, healthcare, and responsibility of a new family member for their entire lifetime, then please consider pet adoption. It's one of the most beautiful ways to circulate love oxygen.

Mikki Moon Star

Made in the USA
Middletown, DE
21 October 2024

62999107R20146